Popular Medicines

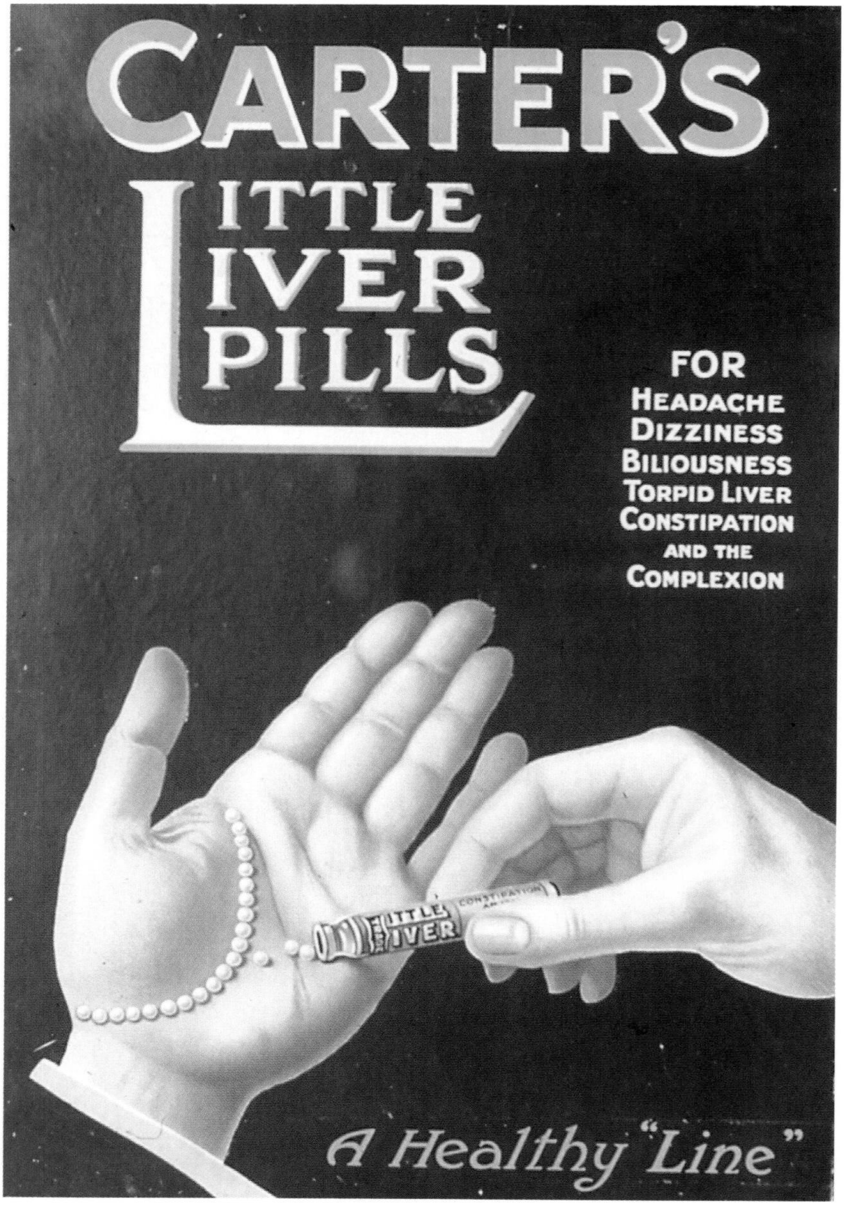
CARTER'S
LITTLE
LIVER
PILLS
FOR
HEADACHE
DIZZINESS
BILIOUSNESS
TORPID LIVER
CONSTIPATION
AND THE
COMPLEXION
A Healthy "Line"

Popular Medicines

An illustrated history

Peter G Homan FRPharmS, MCPP
Honorary Secretary, British Society for the History of Pharmacy
and retired community pharmacist

Briony Hudson MA, AMA
Keeper of the Museum Collections at the Royal Pharmaceutical Society of Great Britain, London, UK

Raymond C Rowe BPharm, PhD, DSc, FRPharmS, FRSC
Chief Scientist, Intelligensys UK and Professor of Industrial Pharmaceutics, School of Pharmacy,
University of Bradford, UK

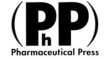

London • Chicago

Published by the Pharmaceutical Press

An imprint of RPS Publishing
1 Lambeth High Street, London SE1 7JN, UK
100 South Atkinson Road, Suite 200, Grayslake, IL 60030-7820, USA

© Pharmaceutical Press 2008

(**PP**) is a trade mark of RPS Publishing
RPS Publishing is the publishing organisation of the
Royal Pharmaceutical Society of Great Britain

First published 2008

Typeset by e-Digital Design, London
Printed in Great Britain by Cambridge University Press, Cambridge
All cover images © Royal Pharmaceutical Society except Carter's Liver Pills © Museum
of Brands

ISBN 978 0 85369 728 2

A catalogue record for this book is available from the British Library

Contents

About the Authors

Peter G Homan FRPharmS, MCPP is a retired community pharmacist and a Member of the International Academy for the History of Pharmacy. Since retirement he has worked as a team member at the Museum of the Royal Pharmaceutical Society and is currently the Honorary Secretary of the British Society for the History of Pharmacy. He has written information sheets for the Museum, articles for pharmaceutical journals and was a contributor to the book *Making Medicines* (Pharmaceutical Press, 2005). Speaking engagements have included Portsmouth University, Thackray Museum, Society of Apothecaries and conferences of the International Society for the History of Pharmacy and the British Society for the History of Medicine.

Briony Hudson MA, AMA studied History at Clare College, University of Cambridge, and Museum Studies at the University of Leicester. Having worked for short periods at museums as diverse as Hereford Cider Museum and the Victoria and Albert Museum, she became Assistant Keeper of Social History for Wakefield Museums and Arts, during which time she co-wrote *Liquorice* (2003, WMDC) with Richard Van Riel, Curator of Pontefract. She joined the Royal Pharmaceutical Society as its Keeper of the Museum Collections in September 2002, where she heads the team responsible for collections of around 45,000 objects. She was the editor of *English Delftware Drug Jars* (Pharmaceutical Press, 2006). She was Chair of the Social History Curators Group from 2005 to 2007, and is a committee member of the British Society for the History of Pharmacy.

Ray Rowe BPharm, PhD, DSc, FRPharmS, FRSC recently retired as Senior Principal Scientist AstraZeneca, having worked in product development for both Zeneca and ICI Pharmaceuticals for 32 years. He currently holds part-time positions as Chief Scientist, Intelligensys Ltd and as Professor of Industrial Pharmaceutics, University of Bradford, as well as indulging his passion for the history of pharmacy through membership of his local museum. He has published over 400 scientific papers, reviews and general articles as well as two books covering subjects as varied as tabletting, artificial intelligence, the history of Bile Beans and quotations for the pharmaceutical scientist.

Acknowledgements

The authors would like to thank the following people, who have generously helped with expertise, information and support:

Stuart Anderson

Vicky Holmes and Jayne Grant, Royal Holloway College

Alan Humphries, Thackray Museum

Bill Jackson

Alice Martin, Bridport Museum

Sarah Maultby, York Castle Museum

Robert Opie, Museum of Brands

Gary Paragpuri, *Chemist + Druggist*

Sarah Pearson, Royal College of Surgeons of England

Kitty Ross, Leeds Museums and Galleries

Rod Tidnam, photographer

Paul Weller, Christina de Bono, Louise McIndoe and Linda Paulus, RPS Publishing

The Library and Museum staff at the Royal Pharmaceutical Society have provided invaluable support and assistance

Unless indicated otherwise, images are reproduced with permission of the Museum of the Royal Pharmaceutical Society

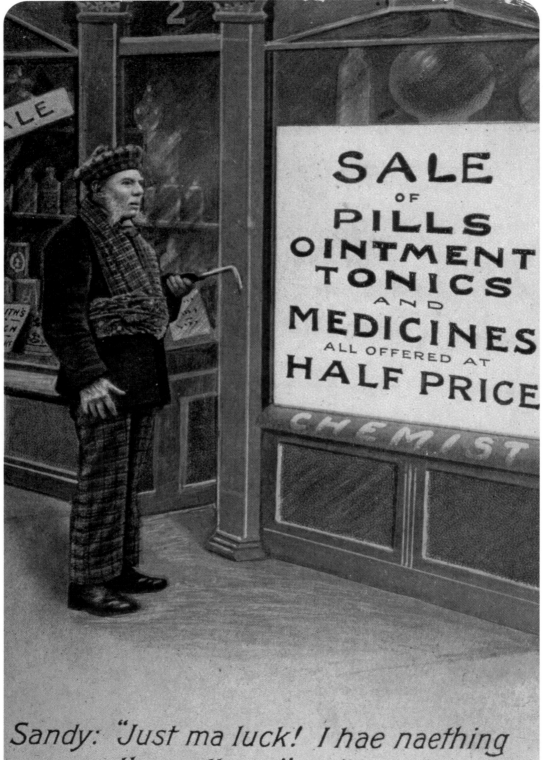

Sandy: "Just ma luck! I hae naething the matter wi' me."

Chapter One
*I*ntroduction

This book looks at a small number of the popular medicines that the public once purchased in the belief that these medicines would cure their illnesses and diseases at prices they could afford. Until the 20th century, doctors' and physicians' fees were out of the question for much of the population.

It is very difficult to date the start of the selling of medicines. It is known that in Britain in the 1100s and 1200s, spicers, who were retail sellers of spices, began compounding and selling medicines. By the end of the 1200s they had combined with the pepperers, wholesale sellers of spices, to form the apothecaries and the first recorded apothecary shop to sell medicines was in 1345. In the 1700s the chemists and druggists appeared, who sold medicines and dispensed prescriptions. In 1841 they, and some of the apothecaries, joined forces to form the Pharmaceutical Society of Great Britain.

Types of medicine

It is important to define the different types of medicine that have been available to the general public.

Nostrum

A nostrum is a traditional product of the apothecary's or chemist's own compounding. The word *nostrum* is Latin and simply means 'ours'. They frequently kept a book of recipes for making up their own nostrums, which would have included medicines, cosmetics and toilet preparations, animal medicines, polishes, inks and dyes. The product would probably bear the compounder's own label. Nostrums were a way of avoiding the payment of medicine tax (see page 4).

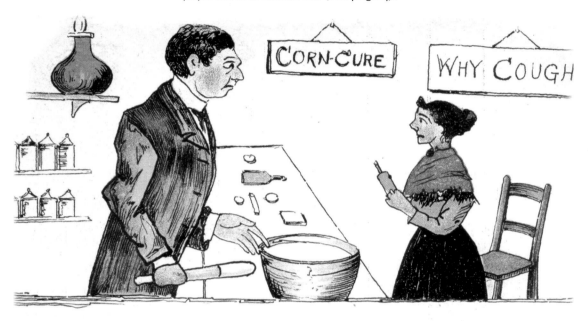

The Chemist explained to his daughter
This stuff that you see in this mortar
You can sell for a cough,
Or take a corn off
By adding a little more water

Quack medicines

Quacks appeared in force during the 1600s. They were also known as charlatans or mountebanks.

The *Oxford English Dictionary* defines a quack as 'an ignorant pretender to skill especially in medicine or surgery, one who offers wonderful remedies or devices'. The derivation of the word 'quack' is probably that it was short for quacksalver or quicksilver, which is mercury and one of the most popular ingredients of the quack's medicine. Another theory is that the word resembles the noise made by the quack as he delivers a presentation to a crowd. The word charlatan is from the Italian *cialare*, to patter, and mountebank from the Italian *monta in banco* – mount on a bench – the position from which a quack would sell his wares.

Quack remedies could contain nothing of medicinal value or perhaps compounds of opium, mercury or antimony. The quack himself would gather a crowd and make wonderful claims for the healing properties of his medicine. In some cases, he would have colleagues planted in the audience who would testify how they had been cured of insufferable ills by this man's medicine. Sales would be made and the team would move on to a new location.

Daniel Defoe in his *Journal of the Plague Year*, 1723, states *'People ran madly after every quack, mountebank and practising old woman who had an antidote or remedy to sell'*.

My Drops and my Pills____Will cure all your Ills.
Printed for & Sold by Bowles & Carver, N°69 in St Pauls Church Yard.

Travelling medicine seller 'Dr Drench' claims 'My drops and my pills will cure all your ills'. (Probably 18th century.) © Royal Pharmaceutical Society

He goes on to mention *'infallible preventive pills'*, *'never-failing preservatives'* and *'sovereign cordials'*.

A century later Oliver Goldsmith, who was a physician, stated *'The English are peculiarly excellent in the art of healing. There is scarcely a disorder against which they are not possessed of an infallible antidote. The advertising professors here delight in cases of difficulty. You will find numbers in every street, who, by levelling a pill at the part affected, promise a certain cure'*.

" by levelling a pill at the part affected, promise a certain cure "

Patent medicines

Patent medicines were deemed respectable because of their association with ancient, royal letters patent, which granted to an individual the sole manufacturing rights for a unique product. To obtain the patent the ingredients of the remedy had to be declared, as well as any manufacturing processes used in the preparation. Patent medicines included Anderson's Scots Pills (*Chapter 2*) and Dr James's Fever Powder (*Chapter 12*).

Proprietary medicine

The *Oxford English Dictionary* defines a proprietary medicine as 'sale of which is protected by patent etc.'. The word proprietary simply means 'owned'.

By contrast to the very formal patenting of medicines, 'secret' formula remedies could cloak their formulas in mystery by simply taking out a trademark. By registering and protecting just the product's name, manufacturers could both discourage outright imitation and capitalise on advertising which had its boom years in the 1800s.

Sale of proprietary medicines was not restricted to Great Britain. Manufacturers were free to export their wares and dealers could import. A number of the medicines featured in this book were produced in the United States of America.

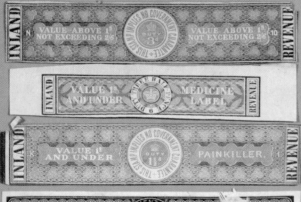

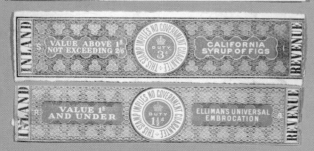

Taxation

The government could see possibilities from the public popularity of proprietary medicines and they became one of the first retail items to be used to raise money by taxation.

In the budget of 1783, a medicine tax was imposed on medicines that were sold by unqualified people – so this excluded doctors and apothecaries. As most sales were through apothecaries, the forerunners to chemists and pharmacists, the tax brought in very little revenue. Non-excluded vendors had to pay a licence fee of 20 shillings or 20/- (£1.00) in London and 5/- (25p) anywhere else. Each medicine had to be wrapped in a piece of paper bearing a government stamp, which stated the amount of duty charged. Adhesive stamps did not appear until 1802. The vendor sent his wrapper to a gentleman called the Commissioner of Stamps who stamped the wrapper and returned it to the vendor.

Penalties for unlawful sales were severe.
- Penalty for selling without licence, 5/- (25p).
- Penalty for selling without proper cover, 5/- (25p).
- Penalty for fraudulently cutting, tearing or taking off such cover, or making use of covers more than once, 10/- (50p).
- Penalty for buying or selling covers used once in order that they may be used again, 10/- (50p).
- Forging any seal, stamp or mark with intent to defraud. Punishment of death without benefit of clergy.

The 1783 Act was replaced by various acts culminating in the Medicines Stamp Act, 1812. Under this act a stamp, representing the tax paid, had to be attached to all manufactured medicines. The sum was dependent on the cost of the medicine. For example, the tax was a penny halfpenny ($1\frac{1}{2}$d) on a medicine with a cost of up to 1/-, such as Elliman's Embrocation, and 3d for medicines costing 1/- to 2/6d such as California Syrup of Figs (see illustration on page 4). This tax was doubled in 1915 as a wartime measure.

In 1940 purchase tax was introduced, which added a percentage of the price of the goods, usually 33% on proprietary medicines, and the Stamp Act was abolished. Value added tax (VAT), which added a percentage to the retail cost, replaced purchase tax in 1973.

Controls over quack and proprietary medicines and their claims as cures were not possible despite laws that were enforced. These laws included the Arsenic Act, 1849, which regulated the sale of that poison, the Pharmacy Act, 1868, limited the sale of medicinal poisons to pharmacists only and the Pharmacy and Poisons Act, 1908, which defined which substances were poisons. None of these acts had any effect on the medicines themselves other than to ensure certain substances were excluded from use, such as arsenic.

Doctors' displeasure

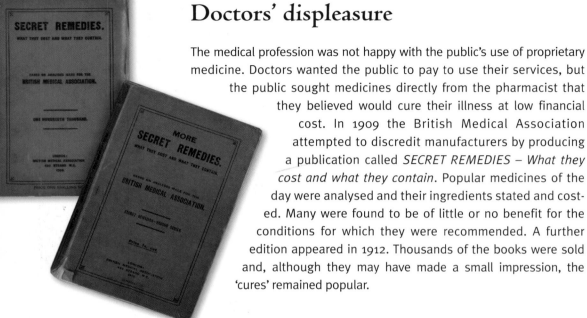

The medical profession was not happy with the public's use of proprietary medicine. Doctors wanted the public to pay to use their services, but the public sought medicines directly from the pharmacist that they believed would cure their illness at low financial cost. In 1909 the British Medical Association attempted to discredit manufacturers by producing a publication called *SECRET REMEDIES – What they cost and what they contain*. Popular medicines of the day were analysed and their ingredients stated and costed. Many were found to be of little or no benefit for the conditions for which they were recommended. A further edition appeared in 1912. Thousands of the books were sold and, although they may have made a small impression, the 'cures' remained popular.

© Royal Pharmaceutical Society

Proprietary Articles Trade Association

Returning to the end of the 1800s, it would have seemed that all was well for chemists and druggists selling these well-advertised proprietary medicines. However this was not the case. There was a great deal of competition from grocers, the emergent multiple drug stores of Jesse Boot and his contemporaries and many other retail outlets, including booksellers. All over the country, companies were cutting the price of proprietary medicines as well as other drugs and household requisites.

The manufacturers were helping the companies. They would offer large discounts on large orders and this discount could be used to lower the retail price. The small chemist and druggist could not afford, or did not have, sufficient sales to be able to buy extra stock and thus compete. He was, in some cases, paying the same price to buy the goods as the multiples were selling the goods. An editorial in *The Chemist and Druggist* in 1893 declared that *'price cutting would see the annihilation of pharmacy proper'* and that, within a few years, *'a few companies would supply all of the pharmaceutical requirements of the country'*.

Enter William Samuel Glyn-Jones. In 1894 he opened a pharmacy as Glyn & Co. in a poor area of East London. Half of his trade was the sale of proprietary medicines, which produced a very low $7^1/_2$% profit as he was having to cut prices to compete with others. He decided that price cutting was a foolish policy and took it upon himself to try to organise retail chemists to press for controlled prices and reasonable margins from manufacturers.

In November 1895 he published a paper called the *Anti-Cutting Record*. His initial run was 5000 copies, which were distributed throughout Britain. He advocated margins of 25% on medicines containing poisons, which only qualified persons could sell, and 15–20% on others. About 600 pharmacists responded who liked the idea. He worked on manufacturers but after six months had the manufacturers of only twelve proprietary medicines on his list. This was enough encouragement to announce in January 1896 the formation of the Proprietary Articles Trade Association (PATA). He kept campaigning, believing that only resale price maintenance would halt the march of the multiples and help the small man survive.

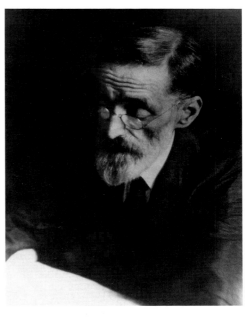

William Samuel Glyn-Jones, 1920s
© Royal Pharmaceutical Society

Below: From *Anti-cutting Record* 1896 © Royal Pharmaceutical Society

Jesse Boot, of Boots the Chemists, was not amused! He was worried that inability to cut prices would mean lost business and was determined to smash the PATA. He and William Day (of Day's Drug Stores) decided to have a mammoth sale of PATA-protected goods. They bought from every source including buying at retail from pharmacists and stored the goods in a disused chapel in London. There was a fire and the goods were destroyed. Some said this was divine intervention. But because of the publicity more small pharmacists realised the dangers and joined Glyn-Jones and the PATA. By 1898 membership was more than 3000.

It was still difficult to persuade manufacturers that resale price maintenance was a good idea. One worry was that chemists would substitute nostrums for

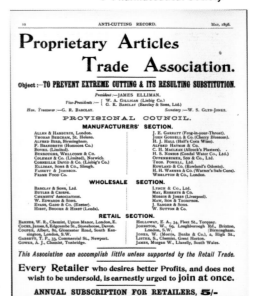

proprietary medicines. The Medicine Stamp Act did not apply to articles of the chemists' own manufacture. In fact, there was a publication that ran for many years, called *Pharmaceutical Joint Formulary*, published by the Pharmaceutical Society, which included formulas for many counter products as well as suggested formulas of many of the proprietary medicines.

The PATA survived. Manufacturers recognised the fact that controlled prices did not mean lower profits. In 1899 Boot and Day abandoned their opposition and gradually company chemists joined the association. Boot realised that resale price maintenance did not mean fixed whole-sale prices and that he could still buy in bulk and make his profits.

Many other trades and manufacturers followed suit and imposed resale price maintenance but it was finally decreed to be against the public interest, and Parliamentary Acts of 1964 and 1976 abolished it on all goods except medicines. On 15 May 2001 the High Court decreed that resale price maintenance on medicines was not in the public's interest and it too was abolished. Later in that year the PATA ceased to function.

Advertising

Proprietary Association of Great Britain

The 1800s saw a huge rise in the number of proprietary medicines. The biggest reason for this growth was the power of advertising. Various media were used, including fliers and newspapers, which often included testimonials (true or false) from 'satisfied customers' who extolled the curative properties of the medicine.

Returning to 1919 and to Glyn-Jones, the government had set up a Department of Health and was about to introduce a bill based on recommendations of a Select Committee on patent medicines. Glyn-Jones thought it essential to set up an association to represent the manufacturers of proprietary medicines. Forty-seven firms met on 2 June 1919 to set up the Association of Manufacturers of British Proprietaries.

At the first meeting on 17 June, it was agreed that members should submit examples of packaging, details of ingredients, place of manufacture and therapeutic and dietetic effects. Firms that dealt with products that might be used as abortifacients or advertised cures for incurable diseases would be excluded from membership. The word 'cure' was allowed provided that it did not claim 'infallibility, certainty or guarantee'. However, the bill did not at that stage lead to an act. The Association continued and, in 1926, changed its name to become the Proprietary Association of Great Britain (PAGB).

A main function of the PAGB has been the control of advertising. In 1924 the PAGB wrote to all newspapers to inform them of its objectives, which in turn led to the newspapers consulting the PAGB on advertising matters, although inconsistency in the type of advertising that they accepted continued. The PAGB formally adopted a Code of Standards of Advertising Practice in 1937, which was accepted by the Advertising Association in 1939 and became the model for rules operated by all of the press organisations in the United Kingdom. The Pharmacy and Medicines Act, 1942, which included controls on advertising of certain diseases, also used the code as a guide.

Today, members of the PAGB still submit advertising and packaging for pre-vetting to ensure the highest standards in press, radio, television and cinemas.

In America, the Food, Drugs and Cosmetics Act, 1938, had similar effects on false advertising and deceptive or unfair practices in the sale of medicines.

National Health

The National Health Insurance Act, 1912, provided free medical treatment to all insured persons. They had to pay for their dependants. Against all predictions this act and the doubling of medicine stamp duty in 1915 had virtually no effect on the sale of proprietary medicines. In 1914 there were 40,000 holders of patent medicine licences; by 1926 this had risen to 60,000 and ten years later the figure exceeded 160,000.

The introduction of the National Health Service in 1948 meant free medicine for all – at least that was the idea. Doctors had the freedom to prescribe any medicine that they wished. Sales of proprietary medicines were depressed and, gradually, many fell from favour and were discontinued.

In 1952 a prescription charge was introduced. Initially the charge was 1/- (5p) per form regardless of the number of medicines and dressings prescribed. This charge was later increased to one shilling per item and then increased year after year. Prescribable proprietary medicines became restricted to those that were not advertised to the public.

In 1984 the Government delivered a heavy blow to the NHS patient. As from the 1 April 1985 only certain medicines would be prescribable on the NHS. The prescribing of a multitude of medicines was forbidden, including cough remedies, digestives, laxatives and analgesics, many of them being household names such as Benylin, Codis, Disprin and Panadol. This is the Black List – a list of all medicines that are *not* allowed to be prescribed on the National Health Service. It was bad news for patients and manufacturers of prescription medicines. However, the combination of the Black List and the escalating prescription charges produced an increase in over-the-counter medicine sales.

Medicines today

In recent years there has also been a great deal of interest in complementary or alternative medicine. Homoeopathy, herbal medicine, aromatherapy, Bach remedies and many more have added to the number of proprietary medicines that are available.

Rather than a box as illustrated on page 11, nowadays one might purchase Regaine Topical Solution for slowing hair loss, one of the increasing number of former prescription-only medicines that are becoming available over the counter in pharmacies. Other such medicines include drugs to reduce gastric acidity, steroids for allergies, antiviral creams for cold sores and tablets to reduce cholesterol levels.

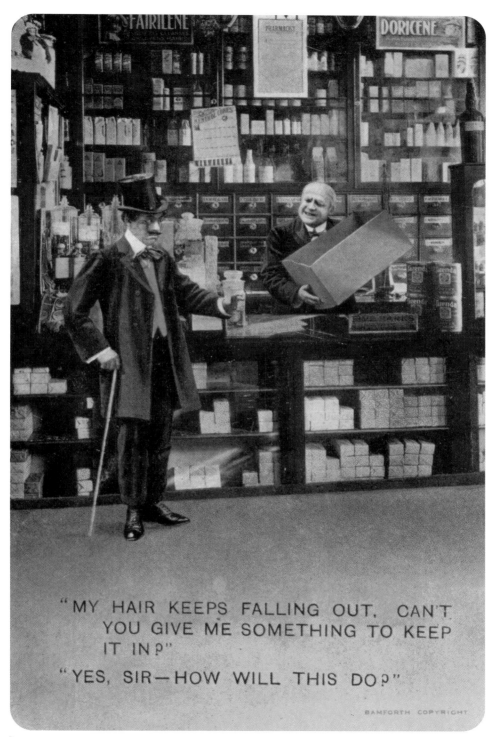

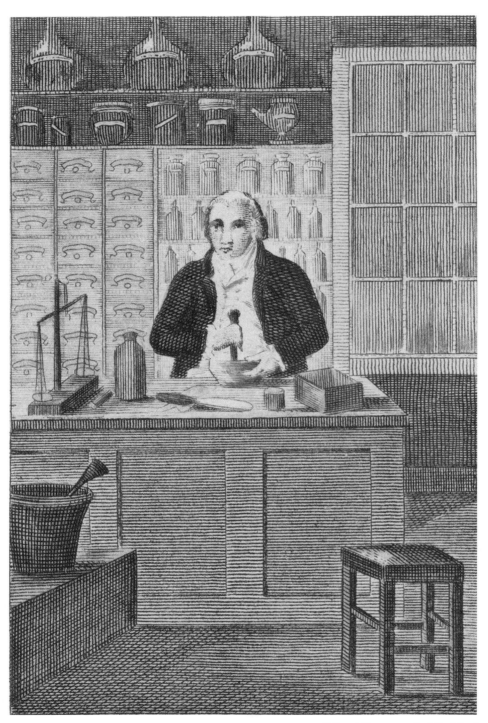

Chapter Two
*A*nderson's Scots Pills

*A*nderson's Scots Pills was a very long-lived product that was popular in Scotland, France and England. Its longevity is thought to be second only to Singleton's Golden Ointment, which is said to have been invented about 40 years earlier.

Dr Patrick Anderson was a Scottish physician who worked in Edinburgh, London and Paris during the 1600s and was described in some of his books as physician to Charles I. He stated that he had obtained a formula for pills in Venice in 1603, which he marketed as Anderson's Scots Pills, Grana Angelica (Angel's Grains). In 1635, he published a treatise entitled *Grana Angelica*, extolling the virtues of these pills.

After Dr Anderson died, the pills were marketed in Edinburgh by his daughter, Katherine Anderson. On 16 December 1686 she declared that she had *'communicated the secret to Thomas Weir, surgeon in Edinburgh, and to no other person'*. In 1694, Dr Weir was granted a patent for the pills by King James II, with *'letters of Certification, etc by King William and Queen Mary'*. Also in 1694 he received *'Testification by the Town Council of Edinburgh'*. The subsequent line of succession of the secret of the pills was:
- from Dr Weir to his widow in 1711
- to their son Alex Weir, 1715
- to his sister, Lilias Weir, 1726
- to Dr Thomas Irving, her nephew, 1770
- to his widow, 1797
- to her son James Irving, 1814.

During and after Mrs Irving's long life (she died aged 99 years in 1837) the pills were made in and sold from the second floor of a house in the Lawn Market, Edinburgh. The property then passed into the hands of a Mr J Rodger who sold his rights to Messrs Raimes, Blanshard & Co. in 1876. They and their successors Raimes, Clark & Co. Ltd (who were wholesale chemists until 1988), carried on marketing the pills until 1916. They donated a sample of the last remaining pills to the Museum of the Royal Pharmaceutical Society in 1956.

A few years after Thomas Weir had taken out his patent, the formula came into the hands of Mrs Isabella Inglish who declared in a bill that she was *'authorised by their Majesties to prepare and publish them at the* Hand and Pen *near the King's Bagnio in Long Acre, London'*. It is said that she actually discovered the formula while working as a servant for Thomas Weir and pirated it. She stated that *'she alone makes Dr Anderson's Grana Angelica or the famous true Scots Pills and no others are genuine'* and accused others of counterfeiting. However, according to Jackson, although the Edinburgh Town Council denounced Isabella Inglish's pills as counterfeit in 1690, they continued to be sold by her and her successors for more than 150 years as the *'True Scots Pills, left to posterity by Dr Patrick Anderson of Edinburgh'*.

© W. A. Jackson collection

An Isabella Inglish advertisement in the *London Gazette*, 8 March to 11 March 1707, declares that:

Dr Anderson's or the famous Scots Pills are faithfully pre-pared only by Mrs Inglish living at the Golden Unicorn over and against the Maypole in the Strand, London. To prevent counterfeits from Scotland as well as any about London, particularly near her habitation, you are desired to take notice that the true pills have their boxes sealed on the top (in black wax) with a lyon rampant and three Mullets argent. Dr Anderson's head between II with his name round, and Isabella Inglish underneath the shield on a scroll.

Her competitors included someone named Mogson who *'pretends to have the Receipt from*

Mrs Katharine Anderson as being intimately acquainted with her in Scotland, and hath had the impudence to counterfeit my printed directions verbatim'. John Gray of the Golden Head, between the Little Turnstile and the Bull Inn in High Hobourn [*sic*] also claimed, in 1699, to make the pills *'according to the doctor's method during his life-time'*. He sealed his boxes with red sealing wax bearing his coat of arms with the words *'Remember you must die'*. Mr Man made and sold the *'True Pills'* at Old Man's Coffee House, Charing Cross in 1703.

The Museum of the Royal Pharmaceutical Society possesses what is thought to be a copy of a flier for the pills that bears a part-copy of a translation of Dr Anderson's *Grana Angelica*. It lists conditions that may be treated and the doses required. It is too long to reproduce in full but a summary follows:

I. *They exceedingly comfort and strengthen the stomach ... purge Choler and Melancholy, but chiefly Phlegm and Waterish Matter ... they comfort the Bowels and remove all obstructions in those parts.*

II. *They strengthen the Head and Senses ... Giddiness and the Megrim ... as they comfort and purge the Stomach, they do the like to the Head and Heart.*

III. *They are beneficial to all Diseases of Women ... may be taken by Women with Child*

IV. *They kill all kinds of Worms ...*

V. *In Women and Child ...have always some of these pills for neither Clysters nor Suppositers are so convenient ...*

TRUE SCOTS PILLS,
LEFT TO POSTERITY BY
Dr. PATRICK ANDERSON, of Edinburgh,
PHYSICIAN TO HIS MAJESTY KING JAMES, I.
AND CONSTANTLY USED AS HIS ORDINARY PHYSIC BY
KING CHARLES, II.

I.—THEY exceedingly comfort and strengthen the Stomach ; restore the lost appetite ; purge Choler and Melancholy, but chiefly Phlegm and Waterish Matter ; cleansing it of all putrid, gross, and thick humours ; they comfort the Bowels, and remove all Obstructions in those parts.

II.—They strengthen the Head and Senses, chiefly those of Hearing and Sight, whose Weakness and Pain they remove ; and help Giddiness and the Megrim ; and as they comfort and purge the Stomach, they do the like to the Head and Heart and, being mixed with other Physic, correct its malignity, and make it unhurtful to the Stomach, and are therefore to be preferred to all other gentle and easy Medicines.

III.—They are beneficial in all Diseases of Women, proceeding from Coldness, change of Constitution, for they safely and easily purge without Pain or Gripping. They may be taken by Women with Child without any hazard of miscarrying, taking one Pill at night after Supper.

IV.—They kill all kinds of Worms that are bred in Men, Women, and Children ; and by frequent use of these Pills, prevents their return.

V.—In Women with Child, great care should be taken to prevent costiveness, which is sure to augment their Pains in travail ; to avoid which, have always ready some of these Pills, for neither Clysters nor Suppositers are so convenient in the time of delivery, afford great help without any danger.

VI.—They gently purge and throw out by stool all Choler seated in the Stomach and Bowels ; therefore are given to those who are tormented with the Headache, occasioned by noisome Vapours that continually ascend thereunto from the Stomach. And, for the same reason, they are given to those who by growth of Choler are continually thirsty, and have their mouth and tongue always dry, and find a heat and loathing with an overturning in their Stomachs. They are also given to those that are against nature overmuch pale, and who have need to be delivered of superfluous Humours of the body.

VII.—They hinder the procreation of many diseases and the corruption of the food, and defend the body against Surfeit in Eating and Drinking, which frequently after Sleep beget crude Humours ; and are a sovereign help for the Gravel, Scurvy, Cholic, Dropsy, Green Sickness, and Palsy, by taking one every night.

VIII.—If the Head, subject to defluctions, keepeth intelligence with a moist and Foaming Stomach, and threatens the joints with a deluge, these Pills will stop their stream, that they who will use them frequently will be free from Gout and all other diseases of the joints, as also inward and outward Rheumatism.

IX.—They are extremely useful to all *seafaring persons*, especially in *long voyages*, who by taking one, two, or three of these Pills at night, are kept from *costiveness*, which is the *cause of most sickness at sea*, and preserved from *scurvies*, *pestilential fevers*, and other *malignant distempers* frequent in Foreign Countries. They are also of great service before drinking the Tunbridge and other Medical Waters, and are an excellent preparation for Sea-bathing.

X.—They may be used at pleasure, late or early, before or after meat ; being taken after supper, defend the head from Vapours and Fumes that arise in the night. They are taken any time or season, without confinement or hindrance of business, or regard to diet. The dose is from three to six Pills, according as the constitution is ; some weak constitutions, that are easy to purge, may take but one going to bed at night, three of four times a month or week, as necessary, or the temper of the body requires. They give not many stools, nor do they act violently or suddenly, but begin to purge about twelve hours after they are taken—sometimes in a shorter or longer time. With some the first dose operates not at all, although the dose from three Pills and upwards, taken some days together, operates with the greatest facility, whether in summer or winter.

XI.—They are of so easy and innocent operation, that they may be given to a child or very old person with the greatest safety, and the most delicate persons, who cannot take other purgatives, may easily take these. They are an enemy to most diseases, and a friend to the noblest organs of the body, and so much known and approved in these nations, that none who have once tried them, and found the good effect thereof, will be without them. And if such as desire to live long and healthful lives, every night take one of them after supper, they will soon find the benefit of them. They are exceedingly good for those oppressed with the wind in the Stomach.

XII.—Though there be few or none in these KINGDOMS and AMERICA, &c., but know the use and excellency of Doctor ANDERSON's ANGELICAL PILLS, yet perhaps many are ignorant of the dangerous ABUSE they are liable to, by unskilful persons COUNTERFEITING them ; for the future, it is thought fit to signify that the *true Pills* are prepared from the Doctor's original Receipt by authority as above, and that on every box there is a stamp affixed, agreeable to Act of Parliament, with a black seal, representing the Doctor's coat of arms, which may be relied on as *Genuine*.

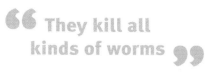
" They kill all kinds of worms "

VI. They gently purge and throw out by stool all Choler in the Stomach and Bowels.

VII. They hinder the procreation of many diseases ... defend the body against Surfeit in Eating and Drinking, which frequently beget crude Humours; and are a sovereign help for the Gravel, Scurvy, Cholic, Dropsy, Green Sickness and Palsy.

VIII. If the Head, subject to defluctions, keepeth intelligence with a moist and Foaming Stomach ... these Pills will stop their stream ... be free from Gout and all other diseases of the joints, so also inward and outward rheumatism.

IX. ... extremely useful to all seafaring persons, especially in long voyages ... kept from costiveness which is the cause of most sickness at sea, and preserved from scurvies, pestilential fevers and other malignant distempers frequent in Foreign Countries.

X. The dose is from three to six Pills ... any time or season, without confinement or hindrance to business ...

XI. They are of so easy and innocent operation, that they may be given to a child or very old person ... an enemy of most diseases.

It ends with a warning about counterfeit preparations

Formula, 1824

Aloes Barbadensis (Barbadoes aloes)	787 parts
Saponis (soap)	131 parts
Colocynthidis (colocynth)	33 parts
Cambogiae (gamboge)	33 parts
Olei Anisi (aniseed oil)	16 parts

The original formula, according to Comrie, contained around 40 ingredients and took about four days to produce using various processes of mixing, steeping, boiling and straining. According to Jackson, the earliest published formula seems to be one that was deposited in the Rolls House in Edinburgh, but has not been traced in recent years. The earliest that Jackson had found was published by the Philadelphia College of Pharmacy in 1824.

Beasley, in 1854, stated that they were *Pilulae Andersonis* of the French pharmacopoeia, which contained only aloes, gamboge and aniseed oil. He then gave four other published formulas, which included the Philadelphia College formula; one containing Barbadoes aloes, jalap, soap, aniseed oil and tincture of aloes; another containing Barbadoes aloes, jalap, powdered aniseed and ivory black; and a fourth containing Barbadoes aloes, black hellebore, jalap, potassium bicarbonate, aniseed oil and syrup of buckthorn.

Pharmaceutical Formulas, 1898, described Anderson's Scots Pills as follows:

> *The original pills are well represented by pil. aloes et myrrhae, B. P., which (saving excipient) contains the same ingredients as those mentioned in a copy of the original document deposited in the Rolls House. American and continental formulas more resemble that for pil. cambogiae co., B. P., but anise is used as the flavouring.*

Formula, 1898

Pulv. aloes bbds. (Barbadoes aloes)	1 ounce
Pulv. cambogiae (gamboge)	1 ounce
Pulv. saponis (soap)	2 drachms
Pulv. glycyrrhiz. (liquorice)	2 drachms
Ol. Anisi (aniseed oil)	20 drops
Syrupi (syrup)	a sufficient quantity

As with other proprietary medicines of the time, we have a very popular pill. It was claimed to possess remarkable curative properties for a large number of medical conditions but was, in common with many others, essentially a laxative. Myrrh was added as a 'stimulant tonic' to stimulate appetite and generally make the patient feel better. Aniseed oil was for flavouring. The gamboge was to expel intestinal worms.

The Author acknowledges the heavy reliance on the article by WA (Bill) Jackson; *Grana Angelica:* 'Patrick Anderson and the True Scots Pills', published in the *Pharmaceutical Historian* in December 1987, volume 17, number 4, pages 2—5.

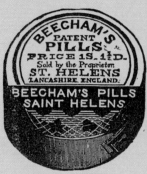

Chapter Three
Beecham's Pills

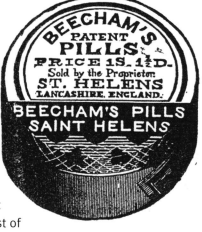

On 30 May 1998, SmithKline Beecham, into which Beecham Proprietary Medicines had evolved, quietly announced that Beecham's Pills were to be discontinued, 'as part of an ongoing rationalisation process'. Thus ended a continuous period of over 150 years during which Beecham's Pills were rarely far from the public's notice, through extensive advertising in magazines, on railway hoardings and on television. Few products had such a high profile as Beecham's Pills, and even fewer played such a critical part in the foundations of what was to become one of the largest of global pharmaceutical corporations.

Thomas Beecham was born of poor parents in the village of Curbridge in Oxfordshire in 1820. He had four sisters and two brothers. At the age of eight he became a farmer's boy earning 18d ($7^1/_2$p) per seven-day week and continued in this employment for ten years. It was while looking after his master's animals that he took an interest in country lore and learned about herbs. His interest in remedies began in his teens, and at the age of 20 he transferred his activities to the newly industrialised areas of Lancashire (in the Wigan area) where he became a market trader. He had a metal stencil made describing himself as 'Chemist, Druggist and Tea Dealer' and a licence, dated 1847, permitting him to sell medicines. By 1842 Beecham had developed his own remedies including Golden Tooth Tincture, Royal Toothpowder, Female's Friend and his famous Beecham's Pills. He began touring the surrounding towns selling his

Left: Reproduced with permission from *The Chemists' and Druggists' Diary*, 1906

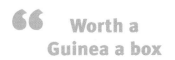

product at markets, particularly St Helens market, where he would sell Beecham's Pills for 6d (2¹/₂p) per box. He also had premises in Milk Street, St Helens, where he set up a mail order business and advertised in the papers *'one box sent post free for eight stamps to any address'*.

The product was immediately successful, and Beecham had to move to successively bigger premises in order to cope with demand. In 1858 he moved his business to St Helens in Lancashire, and opened his first factory. In 1847 he had married a Welsh girl, Jane Evans, who helped him during the Wigan days. In 1875 his staff included his son Joseph as business manager. By then they had started to export to Africa and Australia. There was, of course, no National Health Service in those days but Beecham's employees were given a medical on joining the company and for one penny per week, if ill, were treated in their homes and guaranteed their jobs on recovery.

Beecham's first advertisement was in the *St Helens Intelligencer*, 1859:

> *Worth a Guinea a Box*
> *One trial will convince you that BEECHAM'S PILLS are the best in the world for bilious and nervous disorders, wind and pain of the stomach, headache, giddiness, fullness and swelling after meals, drowsiness, cold chills, loss of appetite, shortness of breath, etc, etc.*

" **Worth a Guinea a box** "

A testimonial from a Mr Mason, boot and shoe maker of Gosborne followed:

> *Sir; about five years ago my wife became afflicted with that distressing complaint, wind and pain of the stomach, and through the violent attacks of spasms she was reduced so low in strength as not likely to recover. She tried many things but all failed to do her good, but to our great joy one box of your pills perfectly cured her.*

Owing to the rapid growth of the business, the factory had to be extended two years later by the addition of a new wing. A new, modern factory covering 1600 square yards was built in 1887 at a cost of £30,000. Much of the machinery was due to the inventive skills of Beecham himself. Alterations and additions were made in 1934, 1948, and finally in 1956.

In 1882 Beecham moved to Mursley, Buckinghamshire, his son Joseph taking over and expanding the business. Thomas Beecham himself retired from the business in 1895 after a lifetime spent building it up. From 1893 he lived in Southport but continued to visit the factory frequently after retirement until he died in 1907. He left two sons, Joseph and William. William qualified as a medical practitioner.

Joseph, born in 1848, was keen to develop the business, and was also a strong advocate of advertising, which he raised almost to the level of an art. During this period Beecham's became one of the largest advertisers in the world. In 1888 the business was established in America with a large factory in New York to make pills. Agencies were established in India and other British colonies and, by the time of Thomas's death, Beecham's was the biggest business of its kind in the world. Joseph Beecham died in 1916 aged 68. He had been an alderman, was mayor of St Helens in 1898 to 1899 and had been knighted.

For eight years following the death of Sir Joseph Beecham, the business was carried on by his executors. However, in 1924 a company called Beecham Estates and Pills Limited was formed, which incorporated the Covent Garden Estates which Sir Joseph had acquired in 1914. The business got into financial difficulties, and Covent Garden was sold off. The arrangement bought out the Beecham family, who ceased to have any connection with the business. In 1928 the company became Beecham Pills Limited. This remained the title until 1955, when it became Beecham Pharmaceuticals Limited

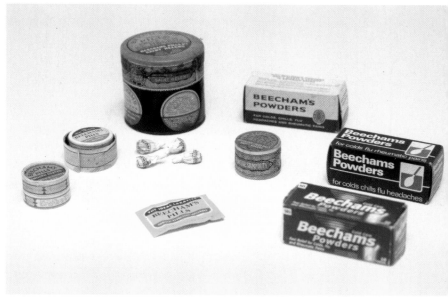

© Royal Pharmaceutical Society

to reflect the growing diversity of the company. It later changed its name to Beecham Proprietary Medicines, part of the Beecham Group.

In 1912 the pills were effectively advertised as a cure-all. *Secret Remedies* reports that:

> *In a circular wrapped round the box it is stated that 'these renowned pills are composed entirely of medicinal herbs,' and cure Constipation, Headache, Dizziness or Swimming in the Head, Wind, Pain, and Spasms of the stomach, Pains in the Back, Restlessness, Insomnia, Indigestion, Want of Appetite, Fullness after Meals, Vomiting, Sickness of the Stomach, Bilious or Liver Complaints, Sick Headaches, Cold Chills, Flushing of Heat, Lowliness of Spirits, and all Nervous Affections, Scurvy and Scorbutic Affections, Pimples and Blotches on the Skin, Bad Legs, Ulcers, Wounds, Maladies of Indiscretion, Kidney and Urinary Disorders, and Menstrual Derangements.*

Much of the early success of Beecham's Pills was down to clever and creative marketing.

Thomas Beecham himself used a variety of techniques to promote his products, initially from a barrow in St Helens market. But the success of the product was down to uncontrolled advertising. His first advertisement was in the *St Helens Intelligencer*. He had adopted the slogan 'Worth a Guinea a Box' from what was said to have been the unsolicited testimonial of one Mrs Ellen Butler.

Thomas Beecham stated his philosophy:

> *It is possible by plausible advertisements, set forth in attractive style, to temporarily arrest the attention of a certain number of readers, and induce them to purchase a particular article. But it is a more difficult matter to ensure their continued patronage. Unless the advertised article proves to be all that is claimed for it not only do the purchasers discontinue its use, but warn others against it as a thing to be avoided.*

Beecham's expenditure on advertising increased from £22,000 in 1880 to over £120,000 in 1891. Fourteen thousand newspapers around the world are said to have carried his advertisements. He produced a reference book for students in 1889 called *Help to Scholars* and distributed over 47 million copies. He published over 20 song-books featuring such

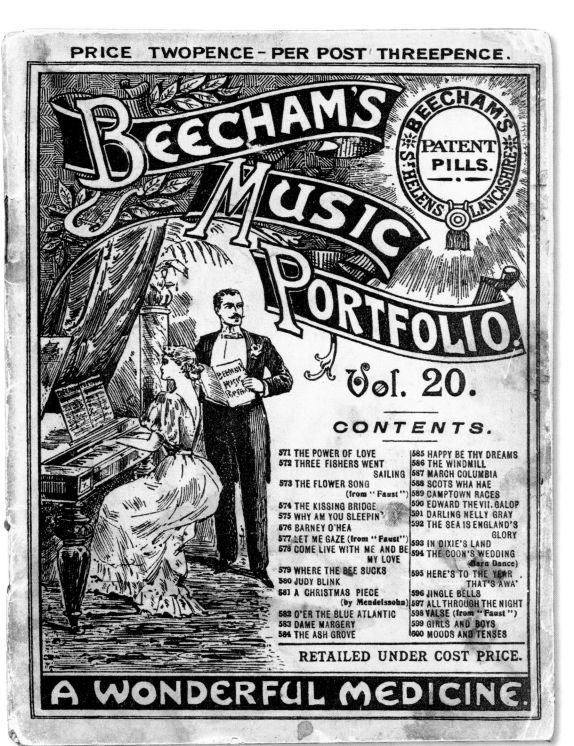

classics as 'Men of Harlech', 'St Helen's Waltz' and the 'Guinea-a-Box Polka'.

Another method of advertisement that Beecham used was the 'unsolicited testimonials', one example being from F Sharp, ship's carpenter of the polar ship *Windward* in 1895:

> *I wish to express my heartfelt thanks to you. I was one of the very few members of the crew of the 'Windward' who did not suffer as a result of one of the most perilous Arctic voyages ever recorded. I did not have one day's illness and I took no medicine but 'Beecham's Pills'.*

Following formation of Beecham Pills Limited in 1928 the company employed two sets of travellers: one for retail chemists, and one for small wholesalers. These methods continued well into the 20th century. A Dr Gorman, recalling his early career in 1985, recalls:

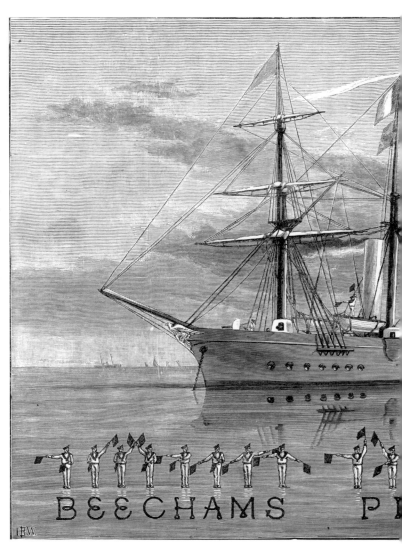

> *I know there was a legend to do with Beecham Pills. A man used to fake a sort of desperate turn on a busy railway station, and then get up and walk away saying 'well, if I hadn't taken 19 Beecham Pills, I'd have been carried off on a stretcher'.*

Humour played an important part in the advertising of Beecham's Pills. Indeed, a number of the early advertisements were drawn by the famous cartoonist, Captain Bruce Bairnsfather. He was the creator of 'Old Bill', devised while he was serving in the trenches during the First World War. An example of his work is an advertising card captioned *'Beauty and*

Health Go Hand in Hand'. The man holds the hand of a beautiful young woman in one hand, and a small, round pill box of Beecham's Pills in the other. Beneath the couple is the slogan '*Take Beecham's Pills: Best for Me, Best for You*'.

In the post war period Beecham's Pills continued to be advertised extensively, in the national press, on cinema screens, on radio and on television. For a number of years the company sponsored the two most popular programmes on Radio Luxembourg, *Take Your Pick* and *Opportunity Knocks*.

Beecham's had begun to diversify at an early stage. Early products included Beecham's Cough Pills and Beecham's Tooth Paste. Beecham's Powders were introduced in 1926, and by 1951 these and Phensic, a painkiller, were already the most important products for Beecham's Pills Limited. By a process of acquisition Beecham's greatly extended its portfolio of proprietary medicines. By the 1990s sales of Beecham's Pills had dropped to the point where their continued production was not viable. Thus ended the life of one of Britain's best-known and long-lived remedies.

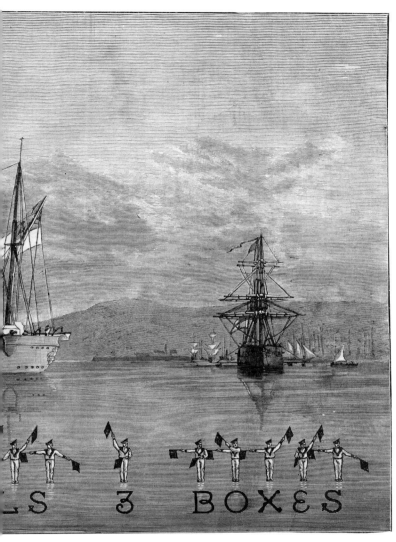

Advertisement from the Illustrated London News, 1890

Beecham's Pills appeared in the chapter on Cure Alls in *Secret Remedies* which recorded that '*a box of these pills, advertised to be worth a guinea, is sold for 1/1¹/₂d* [one shilling and a penny halfpenny]*, and the prime cost of the ingredients of the fifty six pills it contains is about half a farthing* [an eighth of a penny].'

Formula, 1909

Aloes	0.5 grains
Powdered ginger	0.55 grains
Powdered Soap	0.18 grains

Formula, 1977

Each pill contains:

Powdered ginger	20.3 mg
Powdered coriander	4.4 mg
Hard soap	9.7 mg
Aloes	42 mg
Rosemary oil	700 µg
Juniper oil	700 µg
Anise oil	200 µg
Capsicum oleoresin	100 µg
Ginger oleoresin	400 µg
Light magnesium carbonate	2.5 mg

The report contained a detailed analysis of the pills. *'The pills had an average weight of one and a quarter grains. The quantities were approximate and no other ingredient was found.'*

These basic ingredients remained more or less constant throughout the life of the product. The 27th edition of *Martindale's Extra Pharmacopoeia* in 1977 gives the formula of Beecham's Pills.

The identical formula had appeared ten years earlier in the 25th edition of *Martindale*. In the 31st edition (1996) it was stated that the pills contained aloin.

Beecham's Pills first made their appearance in an official publication only in 1993, some 151 years after their first launch. This was in the *British National Formulary* (*BNF*), number 26, dated September 1993, although other Beecham's proprietary medicines had appeared there for several years. They were listed in Section 1.6, Laxatives, as one of many stimulant laxative preparations on sale to the public, but not prescribable on the NHS. Their significant ingredient was listed as aloin. They made their last appearance in the *BNF*, number 35, of March 1998.

The success of Beecham's Pills owed much to the fact that they actually worked. They contained an active ingredient in a sufficient quantity to have an effect. Indeed, the state of the nation's bowels owed much to the efforts of Thomas Beecham over the last 150 years. Beecham's success equally depended on the national obsession with the need to evacuate the bowels on a strictly regular basis.

The price of Beecham's Pills stayed remarkably constant throughout most of their life. In 1915 the price rose slightly from 1/1^1/$_2$d (5^1/$_2$p) to 1/3d (6p) per box: by 1940 it had risen to 1/4d (7p), including purchase tax. At the time of decimalisation (1970) the price was 3/- (15p). Only in the last decades of the 20th century did the price increase substantially. The final retail price, in 1998, of a large pack of 120

Beecham's Pills was £2.72, and for the standard pack of 60 pills the price was £1.87.

One of the most popular anecdotes regarding Thomas Beecham's advertising is that of the hymn books. It is said that a Church of England in South Shields with low funds required new hymn books. The vicar approached Thomas Beecham asking that he might supply them for a low cost if Beecham included a small advertisement. Thomas agreed. When the books arrived the vicar was unable to find any advertisement and concluded that Thomas had made a present of the hymn books. On a Sunday just before Christmas the congregation found that they were singing:

Hark the herald angels sing
Beechams Pills are just the thing
For easing pain and mothers mild
Two for adults one for a child.

It is said that Thomas Beecham denied this story but his representatives were trained to go round humming the tune throughout the country.

The author acknowledges the heavy reliance on the article 'Best for me, best for you – a history of Beecham's Pills 1842—1998' by Stuart Anderson and Peter Homan, published in the *Pharmaceutical Journal* 21/28 December 2002, volume 269, number 7228, pages 921--924.

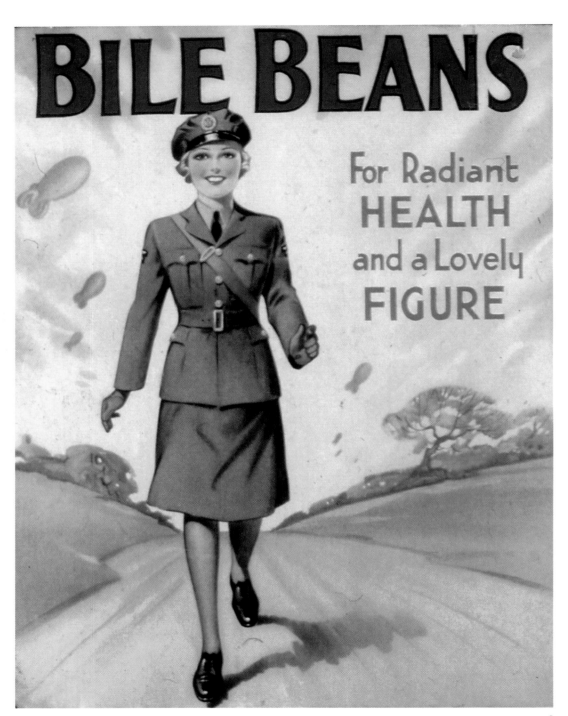

Chapter Four
Bile Beans

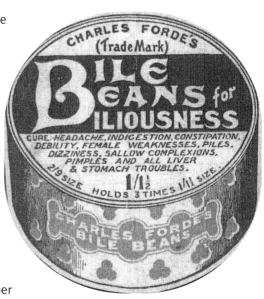

*T*he origin of Bile Beans, arguably one of the most successful products of the early 20th century, stems from a meeting in New South Wales, Australia, in 1896 between Charles Edward Fulford, a Canadian by birth and nephew of George Taylor Fulford, who was then marketing Dr William's Pills for Pale People (Chapter 19), and Ernest Albert Gilbert, an Englishman in his early 20s. Fulford, then 27 years of age had previously spent five years working in a chemist's shop in Brockville, Ontario, Canada, while Gilbert was currently running a stationery and printing business in New South Wales. They agreed to a partnership as medicine and pill manufacturers and launched their first product 'Gould's Tiny Tonic Pills'. Unfortunately this was not a success and in November 1899, Fulford devised a new formulation. He decided upon the name of 'Charles Forde's Bile Beans' – a black ovoid pill packed in a round box.

Under the banner *'Science Uses Nature's Gifts'*, with a picture of a Victorian scientist it was claimed that:

> *Mr Charles Forde, an eminent scientist ... has practically presented a most marvellous medicine as a gift to the human race. He had long been impressed with the superiority of vegetable medicines,*

and devoted himself to the thorough investigation of the properties of roots and herbs peculiar to Australia. After long research he found a natural vegetable substance which acted on the liver and digestive organs in a better way than any medicine known. The best laboratories, the most modern plant, and all the latest scientific methods were requisitioned in the compounding of this substance with other vegetable essences into small beans, which, being unequalled in their operation on the liver and its secretion of bile, were called 'Bile Beans'.

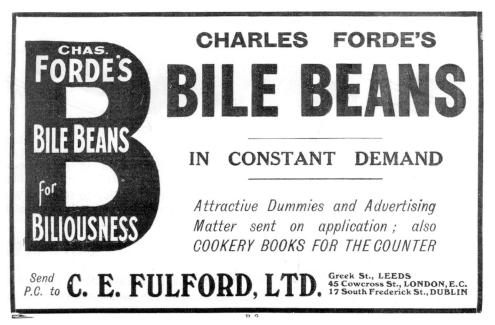

Advertisement reproduced with permission from *The Chemists' and Druggists' Diary,* 1912

At first manufacture was undertaken in Australia but demand soon exceeded supply and manufacture was transferred to Parke Davis and Co., Detroit, USA. At about the same time Fulford opened a factory in Leeds, England. By 1905, agencies selling the product had been set up throughout the world including South Africa, the Philippines, Hong Kong and India. In the UK alone Fulford and Gilbert had spent £300,000 in five years on advertising through sampling and pamphlet distribution. Over 14 million pamphlets were distributed by a workforce of 200 and by 1904 over 2000 chemists were selling the product. It was claimed that the product *'positively cured Headache, Influenza, Scrofula, Piles, Liver trouble, Bad breath, Fulness after eating, Constipation, Lack of ambition, Flatulence, Debility, Female ailments, Pimples, Rheumatism,*

Indigestion, Dizziness, Anaemia, Ulcers, Buzzing in the head, and all Liver and Stomach ailments'.

A cookery book containing 100 recipes for *'homely and economical dishes'* and a collection of printed music containing various compositions for voice and piano *'none too difficult for the average player or singer'* were offered as gifts. Needless to say both contained adverts and information on Bile Beans as well as offering medical advice and publishing endorsements and personal testimonials. A particularly interesting endorsement was one from the scientific journal *Science Siftings* which, after analysing the product, recorded:

> *We have satisfied ourselves that Bile Beans are of purely vegetable origin . . . Our laboratory experiments and practical tests have disclosed to us a valuable preparation . . . excellent for constipation . . . and as a regulator of the liver and bile. Bile Beans increase secretion in the whole of the digestive tract. When employed to relieve constipation they do not—as in the case with so many purgatives—cause after-constipation. There is no griping. They relieve flatulence, sick headache, and biliousness . . . Bile Beans are an excellent family medicine, and we award the Certificate of Merit to the Bile Beans Co. in respect of them.*

❝ we award the Certificate of Merit to the Bile Beans Co. ❞

Inevitably the success of the product attracted imitators and court proceedings were successful in a number of alleged infringement and substitution cases. However, in one celebrated case involving a George Graham Davidson, a chemist in Edinburgh, Scotland, who was selling his own product 'Davidson's Bile Beans', the case went against the partners. They had sought an injunction and claimed exclusive rights to 'Bile Beans' at the Court of Sessions, Edinburgh, in May 1905. The evidence was heard in July but in his judgment published in September 1905, Lord Ardwall refused the interdict saying:

> *There was no such person as Charles Forde, his true name being Fulford. He was not an 'eminent scientist', having had no scientific training and no standing whatever as a chemist or anything else; he never investigated the healing extracts and essences of Australian roots and herbs; he never made any research; he never*

was the discoverer of a natural vegetable substance which had the power of acting in the same way as animal bile; in fact, no substance existed, and no such substance formed the basis, along with other ingredients, of Bile Beans, these beans being compounded by wholesale chemists in America out of the drugs which they had in stock and no one of which had anything specially to do with Australia. There was, therefore, no doubt that their business was one founded entirely upon fraud, impudence, and advertisement . . .

66 their business was one founded entirely upon fraud 99

As regards the exclusive use of the words 'Bile Beans' as a trademark, Lord Ardwall said that the court was bound to take notice of the fact that the words had been used in connection with fraudulent trade and that the complainers' application should be refused. At an appeal in July 1906, the earlier decisions were upheld. Gilbert died soon after the first judgment and Fulford died soon after the appeal. Fulford's and Gilbert's executors and trustees appealed to the House of Lords in the UK but then withdrew before the case was heard. Soon after this, the company changed its name to CE Fulford Ltd with its headquarters in Leeds.

Despite these judgments, the product continued to be sold. In 1912 the pills were priced at 1/1^1/$_2$d (about 6p) for a box of 30, and 2/9d (about 14p) for a box of 90. They were described as *'absolutely unequalled for biliousness and other complaints including anaemia, piles, influenza, despondency, blackheads, and rheumatism'*. It was further stated that the product cured *'fatty and waxy degeneration of the liver, Hob-nailed or Gin-drinker's liver, and the host of ailments having a common origin in impaired digestion, assimilation, and secretion, and in defective working of the excretory organs'*. The pills were *'likewise of estimable service in all the disorders peculiar to women'*, while as a general aperient and tonic they were *'unsurpassed'*.

Up to this point in time nothing had been published as to the formulation of the product, other than a statement *'Bile Beans do not contain a single particle of Mercury, Bismuth, or any other poisonous mineral substances, and are also devoid of Aloes'*. Independent tests by the British Medical Association revealed that there was very clear evidence of the presence of aloin, powdered cardamom, oil of peppermint and wheat flour. There was also evidence, but not conclusive proof, of the presence of extract of colocynth. In fact, this was the formula that was quoted up to the 1930s when the full formula was revealed.

The ingredients read like the pages of a textbook of pharmacognosy and would no doubt have been used in substantiating the 'claims' for the product. At first sight it would appear that the product is a drastic purgative but, in fact, it is more than that. Aloin (aloes barb.), podophyllum and cascara were used as purgatives purely for constipation. Scammony (now called ipomoea), jalap and colocynth were used as hydragogue cathartics which, as well as causing rapid purgation, also removed water, lowering blood pressure and relieving oedema. Leptandrin and soap (saponis) were used as cholagogues to promote the flow of bile (this also potentiated the activity of the scammony and jalap by emulsifying the resins). Cardamom, capsicum, ginger (zingiber) and peppermint oil were used as carminatives preventing griping and flatulence. Gentian was used to improve appetite and stimulate gastric secretion.

Formula 1938

Aloes Barb. (Barbadoes aloes)	6.67%
Res. Podoph. (Podophyllum)	4.42%
Res. Scammon (Seammony)	8.85%
Leptandrin	3.30%
Pulv. Ext. Jalap (Jalap)	8.85%
Pulv. Ext. Coloc. (Colocynth)	2.67%
Ext. Gentian	17.78%
Cascarin (Cascara)	6.67%
Cardam. (Cardamon)	2.67%
Zingib. (Ginger)	10.67%
Saponis Cast. (Soap)	1.65%
Ol. Menth. Pip. (Peppermint oil)	4.42%
Ol. Res. Capsici (Capsicum oil)	0.75%
Ol. Res. Zingib. (Ginger oil)	4.42%
Excipients to	100.00%

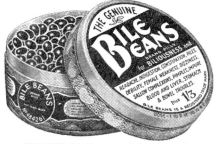

IN BRISK & EVER-INCREASING DEMAND

THE GENUINE BILE BEANS

Bile Beans (Brand Pills) are sold in **6d., 1/3, 3/- and 5/-** sizes. The popular 5/- size contains Bile Beans in 80 penny twists ready for sale; it is very handy for small purchasers.

British Registered Trade Mark (No. 484261).

BECAUSE Bile Beans stock "turns over" so quickly, this well advertised line is one of the most profitable you can handle. National press and broadcast advertising are increasing the demand every day in the year. As their vast popularity proves, Bile Beans remain to-day—the best vegetable pill ever put before the public.

C. E. FULFORD Ltd., CARLTON HILL, LEEDS

In 1930, the product was a brand leader in the laxative market and world sales were over one million pills per day. Claims for the product at this time included *'biliousness and headache, indigestion, constipation, piles, debility, female weakness, dizziness, sallow complexions, pimples, impure blood and liver, stomach and bowel troubles'*.

Advertisement from Butler and Crispe catalogue, 1939
© Royal Pharmaceutical Society

An interesting point of detail on the tin box is the wording *'Bile Beans is a registered trade mark'* – this despite Lord Ardwall's judgment a quarter of a century earlier!

In the early 1940s, the product was extensively advertised in fashion magazines sometimes with the aid of scantily dressed young women *'for inner heath and a lovely figure'*.

An advert under the banner *'How does she keep so slim and lovely?'* stated *'She simply can't help attracting attention with her clear skin, radiant health and slender figure. She keeps in perfect health by taking Bile Beans each night at bedtime'*. It was even implied that the Women's Auxiliary Air Force could rely on Bile Beans to keep them healthy and fit.

Fulford's description of the invention of Bile Beans. From *100 Recipes Cookery Book* **© Leeds Museums and Galleries (Abbey House)**

Science Uses Nature's Gifts.

FROM the very earliest times mankind has endeavoured to penetrate the secrets of Nature. Science owes everything to Nature, and the world is daily benefiting by the remarkable discoveries which Nature reveals to mankind through the researches and experiments of learned and scientific men. One of the most beneficent gifts which Nature has within recent years bestowed upon humanity is undoubtedly the discovery of that wonderful medicine which is now known everywhere by the name of Bile Beans. It has been said that if a man makes two blades of grass grow where only one grew before, he has rendered a service to the world. If this is true, what then must be said of Mr. Charles Forde, an eminent scientist, who has practically presented a most marvellous medicine as a gift to the human race? He had long been impressed with the superiority of vegetable medicines, and devoted himself to the thorough investigation of the properties of roots and herbs peculiar to Australia.

After long research he found a natural vegetable substance which acted on the liver and digestive organs in a better way than any medicine known. The best laboratories, the most modern plant, and all the latest scientific methods were requisitioned in the compounding of this substance with other vegetable essences into small beans, which, being unequalled in their operation on the liver and its secretion of bile, were called "Bile Beans."

The product survived the introduction of the National Health Service in 1948 and was manufactured throughout the 1950s and early 1960s by the same company in Leeds. During this time there were only minor changes to the ingredients; the main one being the removal of leptandrin and soap and the inclusion of sodium tauroglycocholate (presumably as an emulsifier for the jalap and ipomoea resins). This, of course, resulted in the product losing its claim to be purely vegetable in origin. However, much was made of the *valuable new ingredient for disposing of fats which cause flatulence and indigestion*' allowing the product to be 'the family's safeguard against everyday ills'.

In 1964 the company was acquired by Fisons of Loughborough, England, which continued manufacturing the product until its withdrawal in the mid 1980s. During this time the formulation was standardised.

It is interesting to note that although the product is now defunct, an advert for Bile Beans painted on a wall in the City of York some time in the 1940s was recently declared a significant landmark and concern was expressed that any redevelopment of the site should be done without detriment to the advert.

Formula 1964 – 1982	
Cascara dry extract	17.8 mg
Jalap resin	3.09 mg
Peppermint oil	0.89 mg
Ginger oleoresin	1.57 mg
Powdered ginger	12.59 mg
Capsicum oleoresin	0.79 mg
Extract of colocynth	4.97 mg
Powdered aloes	23.4 mg
Cardamom fruit	1.82 mg
Ipomoea resin	4.38 mg
Sodium tauroglycocholate	11.24 mg
Powdered gentian	5.11 mg
Extract of gentian	10.37 mg
Powdered liquorice	14.81 mg

Wall advert © City of York Council www.imagineyork.co.uk. Reproduced by kind permission of Ann Gordon.

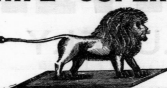

Chapter Five
Burgess's Lion Ointment

*T*here is certainly no dispute over the date and place of the introduction of this product – 1847 in Wandsworth High Street, South London – but there is controversy over the circumstances of the inventor – Edwin Burgess. Company tradition states that Burgess was a jeweller and that he had formed a partnership with a doctor to manufacture and sell the ointment. However in a sworn affidavit in 1892, Burgess's son, Edwin junior, stated *'that his father was originally a hairdresser and had invented the ointment as a hair restorer but found it effectual in curing sores, ringworm and the like'*. He also stated that Edwin senior personally saw to the manufacture of the ointment and composed the first advertisement.

In the latter half of the 19th century, Lion Ointment, with its distinctive trademark, registered in January 1885, was being sold throughout the world. In an advert from 1886 under the banner *'Amputation avoided—the knife superseded'*, the ointment was claimed to:

> **Amputation avoided – the knife superseded**

> cure the worst and most obstinate cases of Ulcers, Abscesses, Cancers, Tumours, Polypi, Carbuncles, Piles, Poisoned wounds of all kinds (including Dog and Venomous Bites), and every form of Eruption and Skin Disease; also Ulcerated and Cancerous Affections peculiar to Females, without the aid of Lancet or Knife. Numbers have been cured after leaving various London Hospitals as incurable, or curable only by amputation.

Left: Reproduced with permission from *The Chemists' and Druggists' Diary*, 1886

The advert also reproduced a number of testimonials and counselled the reader to visit 117 High Holborn, London, to view various cancers, tumours and diseased bones as well as photographs of cases cured by the application of the ointment, all providing proof of efficacy.

In June 1892, Edwin senior, now suffering from 'softening of the brain' was declared bankrupt and the business at High Holborn went into liquidation. After a short but successful court battle with Henry James Deacon who had purchased the goodwill and trademark of the business from the Official Receiver, Edwin junior won the right to manufacture and sell the original formulation. He moved the company to 59 Gray's Inn Road, London, recommenced manufacture and took the business to even greater heights. At its peak the business employed 20 – 30 staff.

A circular enclosed with the medicine in the early 1900s claimed:

> *E. Burgess's Lion Ointment has deservedly become the popular remedy for curing all diseases of the Skin, Old Wounds, Ulcers, Abscesses (including Tuberculous), Tumours, Polypuses, Piles, Fistulas, Shingles, Venereal Sores, Broken Breasts, Bad Legs, Boils, Scrofula (King's Evil), Scorbutic Eruptions, Poisoned Wounds of all kinds, Venomous Bites, Scurf, Ringworm, Itch, Corns, Chilblains, Chapped Hands, Cracked Lips, Cuts, Burns, Scalds, Gatherings in the Ear, Toothache, Earache, Neuralgia, Rheumatism, Gout, Sciatica, Quinsey, Bronchitis, Asthma, Deafness, etc.; also Ulcerous Affections of the Womb, for the treatment of which apply to the Proprietor, personally, or by letter, in all cases free.*

The circular then went on to state that the product had been introduced only after it had been *'practically proved effectual'* and that it was recommended to *'those who are suffering from diseases apparently requiring amputation as it did away with the necessity for the same by drawing in all the cause of the disease from the afflicted part, cleansing the blood and restoring the system to a sound, healthy condition'*.

The ointment could be *'applied with perfect confidence to the most tender skin and as it is entirely free from all poisonous ingredients, a great recommendation for the nursery—for which it is invaluable'*. It is

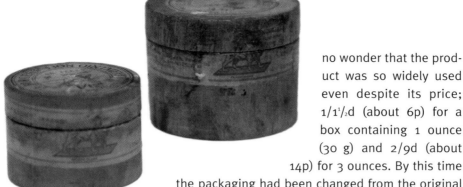

no wonder that the product was so widely used even despite its price; 1/1½d (about 6p) for a box containing 1 ounce (30 g) and 2/9d (about 14p) for 3 ounces. By this time the packaging had been changed from the original greaseproof cardboard boxes to distinctive wooden boxes made from willow.

An analysis of the ointment in 1908 showed its principal ingredients to be lead oleate 13%, resin (colophony) 11% and beeswax 20%, blended with fatty ingredients whose 'identification cannot be placed beyond doubt' although olive oil 12%, water 6% and lard to 100% were suggested. It

© The Chemists' and Druggists' Diary

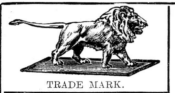

THE LION OF THE DAY.
BURGESS' LION OINTMENT

Others may come and others may go, But Lion Ointment stays for ever.

TRADE MARK.

For over thirty years this preparation has steadily progressed in public favour wherever the use of an Ointment is indicated, its sale is world wide, and the trade mark is protected by registration in all the Colonies, and other countries.

To Chemists it may be considered an addition to their Sundries trade, as nearly all users of same require lint, bandages, antiseptic fluid, or some accessory.

Kept in stock by all Wholesale Houses. Showcards, Counter Bills, &c., direct from the PROPRIETOR—

E. BURGESS, 59 Gray's Inn Road, London, W.C.

is interesting to note that at this time the organic salts of lead combined with colophony were often used as astringents for skin complaints and ulcers. The estimated cost of the ingredients was less than 1d per ounce.

The product remained as such for the next 30 years. Boiled and strained lamb fat was bought from Smithfield Meat Market and willow branches were collected by lorry from Essex, shaved and shaped into boxes using lathes. At this time the business was being run by William, Edwin junior's son, together with his son Reg Burgess. By the early 1940s, adverts had

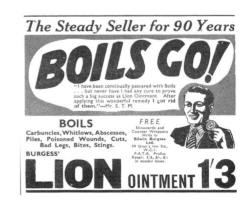

© Royal Pharmaceutical Society

become more focused towards the treatment of boils, carbuncles and abscesses.

In addition, the formulation had been changed, the lead oleate being replaced by zinc oleate, not for the reasons of toxicity but because of the demand for lead for munitions during the Second World War. This change may well have saved the product from extinction as, had it contained lead after the war, legislation would have demanded a withdrawal from the market.

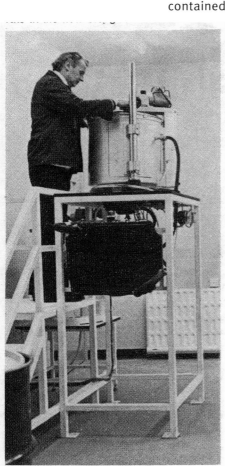

In the 1950s trade began to decline as a result of not only the availability of antibiotics but also the lack of investment in new technology. Although a new plastic container was introduced in the early 1960s, labels were still stuck on by the old, time-honoured and time-consuming method of laying dry labels onto a glued glass plate. In 1954, the company moved from its premises in Gray's Inn Road to a smaller property in north London and thence to Rosomon Street in east London in 1968. From that date, advertising declined, overseas markets were lost and the business dwindled. However the trademarks were maintained and the company still received between eight and ten testimonial letters and inquiries for stockist names every week.

In 1975, the company was bought out by Leo Laboratories and a new manufacturing facility equipped for producing 750,000 units per year established at Slough.

The product, now packed in specially printed jars and with a formulation consisting of zinc oleostearate 5%, rosin (colophony) 5%, anhydrous lanolin 15%, yellow beeswax 5%, yellow soft petroleum jelly 65% and methylated spirits 5% was approved by the Food and Drug

Mr Reg Burgess inspects one of the vats at the new Slough works © *The Chemist + Druggist Magazine*, 1976

Administration for marketing in the USA. New and old markets were re-established with more than 80% of all Lion Ointment produced being exported in orders averaging £1000. In the UK a television cartoon commercial featuring 'Edwin the lion' was introduced

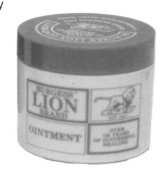

and newspaper advertising increased. Over the next decade the company flourished with sales increasing year on year. In the mid 1980s the company moved into ethical pharmaceuticals with the introduction of Imunovir, an immunostimulant to enhance the body's natural defences to viral disease. Subsequent rationalisations in the late 1980s led to the discontinuation of Lion Ointment.

However, it would appear that the product is not dead. A perusal of the internet has revealed that a version of the ointment is currently being marketed by Feathergills of Hebden Bridge, West Yorkshire. The manufacturers claim that the formulation has been 'slightly modified to make it more easily absorbed' and that the product *will soothe and protect the skin and can be used to treat severely cracked skin, boils, abscesses and draw splinters etc'*. It is interesting to note that Feathergills have retained the original, distinctive lion trademark on the tin.

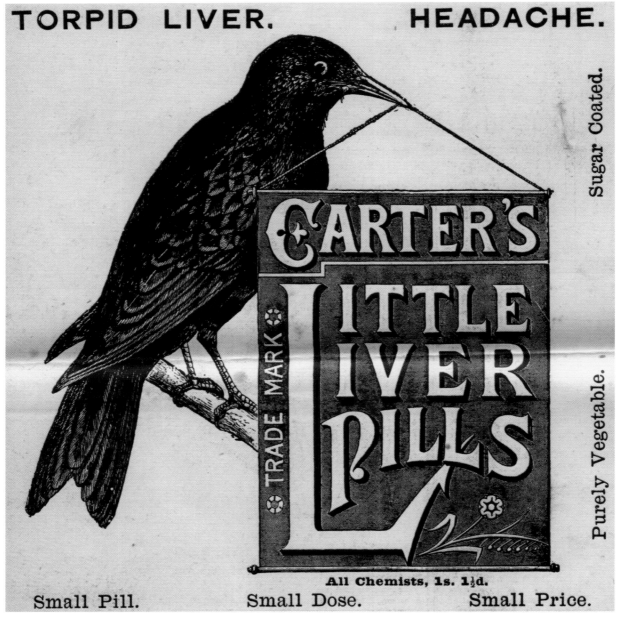

Advertisement from the *Illustrated London News*, 1889

Chapter Six
Carter's Little Liver Pills

Genuinely the invention of a Doctor John Carter from Erie, Pennsylvania, in around 1839, this product is generally associated with the Canadian born entrepreneur Brent Good.

Born in 1837, Good's earliest pharmaceutical experiences were gained in a chemist's shop in Belleville, Ontario, where, from 1851 to 1856, he served his apprenticeship. He then migrated to New York working for Barnes & Co., a wholesaler. In the 1860s Good formed several partnerships, one with the prominent American pill manufacturer William Warner and one with John Carter, who had commenced manufacturing his formulation in 1856, as well as starting on his own account as a wholesale druggist under the name Brent Good & Co. Throughout his life Good was a larger than life character and later on was to become proprietor of the Writing Telegraph Company, The Brent Manufacturing Company, the Conformator Bevel Company manufacturing carpets, the Lyceum Theatre Company in New York and a director of the Franklin National Bank of New York.

MR. BRENT GOOD.

Good purchased the Carter trademark and formulation and became sole proprietor of the Carter Medicine Company in 1889. As a result of extensive advertising costing several millions of dollars the product became a brand leader. Adverts under the banner '*SICK HEADACHE POSITIVELY CURED BY CARTER'S LITTLE LIVER PILLS*' with the statement '*We mean cured, not merely relieved . . . there are no failures and no disappointments*' were commonplace. In addition the product was claimed to cure:

> *all forms of Biliousness, prevent Constipation and Dyspepsia, promote Digestion, relieve distress from too hearty eating, correct Disorders of the Stomach, Stimulate the Liver, and Regulate the Bowels. They do this by taking just one little pill at a dose. They are purely vegetable, do not gripe or purge, and are as nearly perfect as it is possible for a pill to be.*

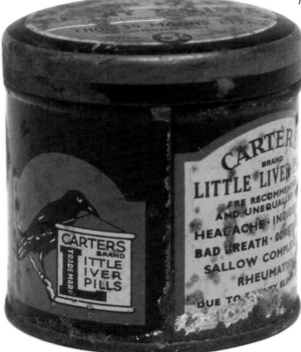

© **Royal Pharmaceutical Society**

By 1886, Good had introduced his pills into the UK using John Morgan Richards as importer. He had met Richards as a fellow employee at Barnes & Co., and Richards subsequently set up a company in London importing American patent medicines. The pills were manufactured in bulk in New York, shipped in bulk to the UK and then packaged in phials of 40 pills under the Carter Medicine Company trademark at 46 Holborn Viaduct, London. The pills were sugar coated, containing podophyllum resin (0.0625 grains), Curacao aloes (0.25 grains), powdered liquorice root (0.00238 grains), powdered acacia (0.006 grains) and wheat starch (0.017 grains).

In the UK the pills were also promoted for 'torpid liver' as well as *'A perfect remedy for Dizziness, Nausea, Drowsiness, Bad Taste in the Mouth, Coated Tongue, Pain in the Side, etc.'.* They were also claimed to *'give the clear eye and bright-coloured complexion of perfect health and beauty'.*

Simple rhymes were used in adverts, for example, preceding a list of complaints, would appear:

> *A Little List of Little Ills*
> *Cured by Carter's Little Liver Pills.*

And often at the bottom of a newspaper advert would appear:

Carter's Little Liver Pills
Cure all Liver Ills.

Customers were invited to send for a free 32-page, illustrated pamphlet entitled *Mr Crow* or *The Rook's Progress*. The reason why these black birds were chosen for the trademark remains a mystery but they were effective. It is interesting to note that the product was one of the very few in the UK at the time that seriously dented the enormous consumer goodwill then enjoyed by Beecham's Pills.

Good was very protective of his product and trademark and treated counterfeiters and pirates of his trademark with contempt. In an interview with *The Chemist and Druggist* in 1896 he stated:

They're a pest, these fellows, both on this side and in the States. And, mind you, I will say this for England: it's easier to get justice here than at home. In America we have to prosecute under a different law in each State. In some sections we can lock 'em up. I imprisoned nine pirates in Illinois within the past few years.

He thought '*no mercy should be shown to men who try to enrich themselves by trading on another's brains and enterprise*'. In later adverts his signature was appended to prove authenticity.

During the First World War a postcard was produced, notable in that it combined

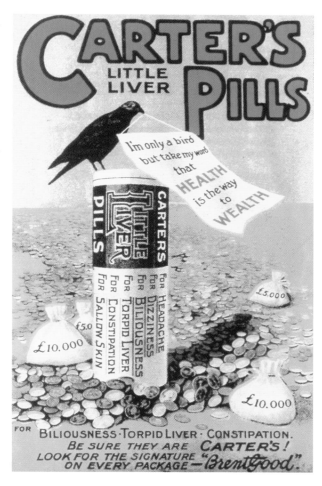

Above and below: © Museum of Brands

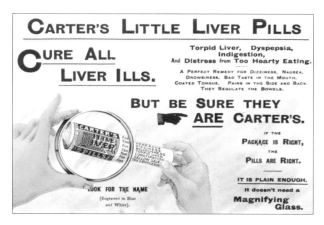

product advertising with a strong patriotic message. Below the flags of Belgium, Russia, Great Britain and Japan under the banner '*Carter's Little Liver Pills For Active Service*' is a picture of a man stripped to the waist (presumably an army recruit) with a suited man (presumably a doctor). The claim was '*for the keen eye of Perfect Health*'. The special free offer at the base of the card was six postcards of historic buildings obtainable by sending an outside wrapper from a phial of the pills.

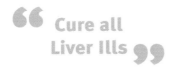
Cure all Liver Ills

In the mid 1920s posters featuring Broadway actresses were used to advertise the product, the viewer being asked to '*Note the sparkling eyes and clear glowing skin after taking Carter's Little Liver Pills for a sick stomach and headache*'.

Brent Good died in 1935 but the product continued as before but was sold in the UK by Thomas Marns Ltd of Caxton Street, London.

In the 1960s the product was sold by Pretested Products Ltd, Rickmansworth. In the 1970s the product was reformulated with each pill containing the laxatives phenolphthalein (16 mg) and aloin (8 mg) and manufactured by Carter-Wallace. After a number of court cases the company abandoned the word 'liver' renaming the product Carter's Little Pills. In April 1992 the pills were withdrawn from the list of products that could be prescribed under the NHS schedules. The product containing bisacodyl is still available in Canada for bowel evacuation and constipation.

Chapter Seven
Clarke's Blood Mixture

*I*n the mid 1800s, the makers of any kind of 'medicine' found little difficulty demonstrating that almost any disease could arise from a part of the body that their own particular nostrum professed to benefit. It was, of course, particularly easy to connect a wide variety of diseases to the condition of the blood. The brand leader of the 'blood mixtures' on sale at the time was Clarke's World-Famed Blood Mixture, invented by Francis Jonathan Clarke and later packed in moulded, cobalt-blue, glass bottles embossed with the product name.

Clarke was born in Lincoln, England, in 1842. At the age of 19, after a short apprenticeship in Mansfield and experience in dispensaries in Lincoln, Kingston-on-Thames and London, he opened his first shop in Newland, Lincoln, and started selling his blood mixture. His business prospered and within a few years he was able to purchase premises in the High Street, Lincoln, and launch his product nationwide. He invested heavily in advertising spending some £15,000 in the first year. Despite being £7,000 in debt, he continued to invest and by the end of the second year he had broken even. Success for his blood mixture was assured and for the next 20 years his sales increased year on year. It is recorded that in this time he spent more than £20,000 per annum on printing ink alone.

© *The Chemist + Druggist Magazine*, 1888

Clarke was very popular and noted for his kindness and generosity. He gave liberally to the poor of the city and took great care of his staff. He was elected mayor of Lincoln four times and was even offered the position for a fifth time in 1886 but declined the honour. He fell ill in 1887 and moved to Bournemouth in the hope that the sea air would help his failing heart and lungs. He died there on 28 January 1888. At his funeral the crowds lined the streets.

© The Chemist + Druggist Magazine, 1878

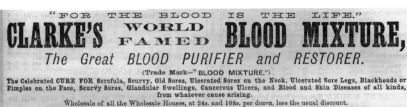

"FOR THE BLOOD IS THE LIFE."

CLARKE'S WORLD FAMED **BLOOD MIXTURE,**

The Great BLOOD PURIFIER and RESTORER.

(Trade Mark—"BLOOD MIXTURE.")

The Celebrated CURE FOR Scrofula, Scurvy, Old Sores, Ulcerated Sores on the Neck, Ulcerated Sore Legs, Blackheads or Pimples on the Face, Scurvy Sores, Glandular Swellings, Cancerous Ulcers, and Blood and Skin Diseases of all kinds, from whatever cause arising.
Wholesale of all the Wholesale Houses, at 24s. and 108s. per dozen, less the usual discount.

Sole Proprietor, **F. J. CLARKE, CHEMIST, LINCOLN, ENGLAND.**

Counter Bills and Posters, with Name and Address, also Show Cards, on application. Printed matter supplied in any Language for Foreign Agents.
CAUTION.—Mr. CLARKE will take immediate proceedings against all persons pirating his Trade Mark, Labels, Wrappers, Bills, or Advertisements or in any way infringing his rights.

"FOR THE BLOOD IS THE LIFE."

CLARKE'S WORLD FAMED **BLOOD MIXTURE,**

The Great BLOOD PURIFIER and RESTORER.

(Registered Trade Mark—"BLOOD MIXTURE.")

The Celebrated CURE FOR Scrofula, Scurvy, Blood and Skin Diseases, and Sores of all kinds.
Wholesale of all the Wholesale Houses, at 24s. and 108s. per dozen, less the usual discount.

Sole Proprietors, **THE LINCOLN & MIDLAND COUNTIES' DRUG COMPANY, LINCOLN.**

Counter Bills and Posters, with Name and Address, also Show Cards, on application. Printed matter supplied in any Language for Foreign Agents.
CAUTION.—The Proprietors will take immediate proceedings against all persons pirating their Trade Mark, "Blood Mixture," Labels, Wrappers, &c., or Advertisements, or in any way infringing their rights.

© The Chemist + Druggist Magazine, 1884

After Clarke's death, his business was put in the hands of executors and his blood mixture continued to be manufactured by the Lincoln and Midland Drug Company. Although the product range was extended to include aperient pills, skin lotion, salves and medicated soap, blood mixture remained as the most well-known and popular product.

An advert from 1878 under the headline '*for the blood is the life*' claimed that the product '*is warranted to cleanse the blood from all impurities, from whatever cause arising. For Scrofula, Scurvy, Sores of all kinds, Skin and Blood Diseases, its effects are marvellous*'. A pamphlet enclosed with the medicine in the early 1900s claimed:

> *No matter what the symptoms may be, the real cause of a large proportion of all disease is bad blood. Clarke's World-famed Blood Mixture is not recommended to cure every disease; on the contrary there are many that it will not cure; but it is a guaranteed cure for all blood diseases . . . It never fails to cure Scrofula, Scurvy, Scrofulous Sores, Glandular Swellings and Sores, Cancerous Ulcers, Bad Legs, Secondary Symptoms, Syphilis, Piles, Rheumatism, Gout, Dropsy, Black-heads or Pimples on the Face, Sore Eyes, Eruptions of the Skin and Blood, and Skin Diseases of every description.*

"**for the blood is the life**"

In 1895, the editors of *Exposures to Quackery* were very critical of these claims. Quoting an analysis of an eight-ounce bottle of the mixture in 1875 by Dr Alfred Swaine Taylor FRS, who found the ingredients to be iodide of potash (64 grains), chloric ether (4 drachms), potash (30 minims solution) and water coloured with burnt sugar, they suggested that, at the stated doses, patients would display iodism – a condition resulting in inflammation of the mucous membranes of the eyes and nose, salivation, purging and nausea.

Advertisements from the early 1900s expanded earlier claims and also refer to the '*thousands of testimonials from all parts of the world*'. It is interesting to note that the editor of *The Family Doctor* was obviously convinced by this evidence for he writes '*We have seen hosts of letters bearing testimony to the truly wonderful cures effected by Clarke's Blood Mixture. It is the finest Blood purifier that Science and Medical Skill have brought to light; and we can with the utmost confidence recommend it to our subscribers and the public generally*'.

Other than the analysis reported in *Exposures to Quackery* very little was known about the formula for the mixture. It was always claimed that '*the mixture is pleasant to taste and warranted free from anything injurious to the most delicate constitution of either sex*' and was to be taken '*about half-an-hour after meals*' at doses depending on the age and sex of the patient: '*one tablespoonful four times a day for adult males, one tablespoonful three times a day for adult females, two teaspoonfuls three times a day for children*

THE CHEMISTS' AND DRUGGISTS' DIARY, 1901   355

"For the Blood is the Life."

CLARKE'S BLOOD MIXTURE

THE WORLD-FAMED BLOOD PURIFIER AND RESTORER.

Trade Mark—"*BLOOD MIXTURE*."   Registered No. 3275.

THE CELEBRATED CURE FOR

SCROFULA, SCURVY, ECZEMA, BAD LEGS, ULCERS, PIMPLES, BLOTCHES, SORES, AND ALL SKIN AND BLOOD DISEASES.

Wholesale of all the Wholesale Houses.

Counter Bills and Posters, with Name and Address, also Show Cards, on application.

Printed matter supplied in any Language for Foreign Agents.

SOLE PROPRIETORS:—

THE LINCOLN AND MIDLAND COUNTIES' DRUG CO.

LINCOLN, ENGLAND.

CAUTION.—The Proprietors will take immediate proceedings against all persons pirating their Trade Mark, "BLOOD MIXTURE," Labels, Wrappers, &c., or Advertisements, or in any way infringing their rights.

© *The Chemists' and Druggists' Diary*, 1901

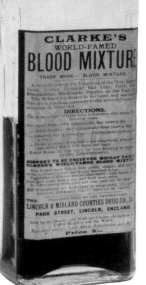

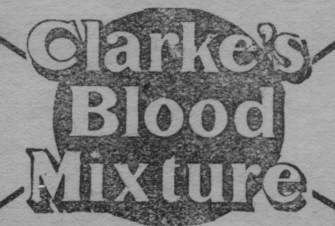

TO SUFFERERS FROM
Skin & Blood Diseases.

For cleansing the blood of all impurities, from whatever cause arising, there is no other medicine just as good as Clarke's Blood Mixture—that's why in so many cases of **Eczema, Scrofula, Scurvy, Bad Legs, Abscesses, Ulcers, Tumors, Boils, Pimples, Blotches, Sores and Eruptions, Piles, Glandular Swellings, Blood Poison, Rheumatism, Gout, &c.,** it has effected truly remarkable cures where all other treatments have failed. Clarke's Blood Mixture has over 45 years' reputation, and the proprietors solicit all sufferers to give it a trial to test its value.

The Editor of the "FAMILY DOCTOR" *writes:*—"We have seen hosts of letters bearing testimony to the truly wonderful cures effected by Clarke's Blood Mixture. It is the finest Blood Purifier that Science and Medical Skill have brought to light; and we can with the utmost confidence recommend it to our subscribers and the public generally."

Clarke's Blood Mixture

HAS CURED THOUSANDS.
WILL CURE YOU.

Sold by all Chemists and Stores—2/9 per bottle.

Advertisement from *The Star Home Doctor*, circa 1904 © private collection

over twelve years of age and from one half to one teaspoonful accord-
ing to age for infants'.

A detailed analysis in 1909 showed it to contain potassium iodide 1.5%,
sugar (partially inverted) 1.2%, alcohol 1.6% by volume and traces of
chloroform and ammonia, and *'a brown colour being given by a small*
quantity of what was evidently burnt sugar'.

Spirit of sal volatile, also known as aromatic spirit of
ammonia, was prepared with ammonia 4% solution,
ammonium carbonate 2%, lemon and nutmeg oil
dissolved in a mixture of alcohol 60% and water 30%.
This mixture would certainly not have had an unpleasant
taste, any bitterness due to the potassium iodide
would have been masked by the syrup and the
chloroform. Both potassium iodide and ammonium
carbonate act as expectorants.

Formula, 1909

Potassium iodide	52.5 grains
Spirit of sal volatile	10 minims
Spirit of chloroform	67 minims
Simple syrup	50 minims
Burnt sugar	q.s.
Water	to 8 fluid ounces

This was the formula that was quoted in all editions of
Martindale, The Extra Pharmacopoeia up to 1935
when the full formula was revealed.

Although containing some of the ingredients found in
1909, others have been added: sodium salicylate as an
antipyretic, potassium bicarbonate to treat acidosis
and potentiate the expectorants, sodium nuclein (a
material prepared by digesting yeast with pepsin and
hydrochloric acid and then neutralising with sodium
hydroxide) to stimulate the production of white blood
cells, neutralising toxins and promoting the healing of
ulcers. Gentian is used to stimulate the appetite and
also as a bitter tonic.

Formula, 1935

Potassium iodide	1.084%
Sodium salicylate	1.304%
Sodium nuclein	0.200%
Potassium bicarbonate	0.865%
Ammonium chloride	0.652%
Conc. compound solution of gentian	0.107%
Chloroform	0.237%
Sp. Vini. Rect. (brandy)	0.237%
Soluble colour	0.498%
Distilled water	94.816%

The dose was one teaspoonful to one tablespoonful and the product
'was highly recommended for blood and skin complaints, eczema,
psoriasis, eruptions, sores, ulcers, ulcerated legs, enlarged glands,
rheumatism, gout etc.'.

The product survived the introduction of the NHS in the UK in 1948 and in the 1950s the formula was modified further, possibly as a result of new legislation. The sodium nuclein and brandy were removed and sarsaparilla included, probably because of its reputation in the treatment of syphilis, rheumatism and psoriasis, thus providing some support for the product claims.

Further minor modifications were made in 1961 when concentrated compound solution of gentian was replaced by concentrated compound infusion of gentian and increased to 0.75%; the sarsaparilla concentration was tripled and the burnt sugar was given as 0.25%. This was the formula that was used until the late 1960s when the product was withdrawn. Unfortunately no claims were supplied for this formulation but no doubt they were certainly modified in the light of the then current UK legislation.

Formula, 1955

Potassium iodide	1.15%
Sodium salicylate	1.85%
Potassium bicarbonate	1.85%
Ammonium chloride	0.70%
Conc. compound solution of gentian	0.25%
Conc. compound decoction of sarsaparilla	0.25%
Chloroform	0.25%
Sacch. Ust.(burnt sugar)	q.s.
Distilled water to	100.00%

Chapter Eight

J Collis Browne's Chlorodyne

*F*ew medicines have had greater impact on the relief of symptoms of disease than Collis Browne's Chlorodyne, a success story that still retains a high volume of sales today and is known in most countries of the world.

THE LATE DR. JOHN COLLIS BROWNE.

The story of J Collis Browne's Chlorodyne involves not one, but two well-known figures, namely Dr John Collis Browne MRCS (1819–1884) and Mr John Thistlewood Davenport, pharmaceutist (1817–1901). The former was the inventor or formulator of the original product and the latter the manufacturer.

Above right: © *The Chemist + Druggist Magazine,* 1874

Above left: © *The Chemist + Druggist Magazine,* 1896

Browne was born in Maidstone, Kent, the son of a Captain in the 13th Light Dragoons. He qualified as Member of the Royal College of Surgeons of England in 1842 and in 1845 was admitted as an extra-licentiate of the Royal College of Physicians in London. In the same year he joined the Army Medical Service as an assistant surgeon in the 98th Regiment. In 1847 his regiment was sent to Dinapore in India at a time when an outbreak of cholera was rampant in Bengal and it is probably at about this time that he first manufactured his 'compound'. Later, Browne was one of the first men in the British Army to serve on the North-West Frontier of India. In 1852 he was back in England at Fort Pitt, Chatham, from where he went to Trimdon, County Durham, to help fight an outbreak of cholera and used his compound with great effect.

In 1856, having left the Army, Browne went into partnership with a chemist, John Thistlewood Davenport of 33 Great Russell Street, London. Davenport, as well as owning a dispensing business, manufactured pharmaceutical chemicals including scale preparations of iron and quinine. It was rumoured that Browne had offered to sell the formula outright to Davenport for £100. Davenport declined until he had satisfied himself of the value of the medicine. In the event the two men made an agreement to share the profits. At that time Davenport was President of the Pharmaceutical Society of Great Britain. This meant that he had to be seen to be very thorough, especially when dealing with a proprietary medicine. He therefore had the medicine well tested by many medical men and it was on their recommendation that he agreed to manufacture the chlorodyne. It has been said that he also made some minor changes to the formulation.

Davenport considered initially that Dr J Collis Browne's Chlorodyne should not be heavily advertised, as was the case with most proprietary medicines, but to rely on its reputation gained abroad and by recommendation. Advertising was confined to professional journals. Later he found that competition dictated that he must increase advertising, but he maintained that all claims made were genuine and that testimonials were not paid for.

Although Browne registered his label at Stationer's Hall, he did not patent the product. This meant others could use the name 'chlorodyne' and cash in on the popularity from advertising. Most notable among the copiers was Freeman who

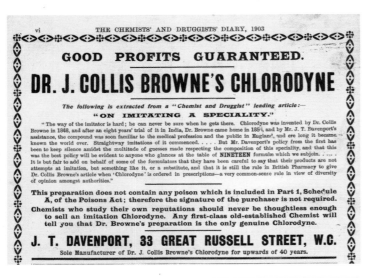

claimed he himself had been the first producer of chlorodyne in 1844 and claimed that Dr Irvine of the Royal Free Hospital recommended his product. Davenport was forced to engage in a war through advertisements in trade papers claiming that *'CHLORODYNE the original and only genuine'* was *'discovered only by Dr J. Collis Browne, M.R.C.S., Late Medical Staff'*.

Browne spent his gains from his share in the profits on inventions, mainly on ships' propulsion and planning a method of raising ships by inflating india-rubber bags with carbonic acid gas, a method that became often used, but he did not patent the process.

Davenport was succeeded by his son Horace Davenport who continued with the company. JT Davenport Ltd continued to manufacture Dr Browne's Chlorodyne until 1980 when production moved to Napp Laboratories, Beverley. Seton Healthcare Group Plc took over in 1995, International Laboratories of Manchester in 1999 and, since 2002, it has been produced by Thornton & Ross Ltd of Huddersfield.

An undated flier advertising Dr J. Collis Browne's Chlorodyne states:

CHLORODYNE is admitted by the profession to be the MOST

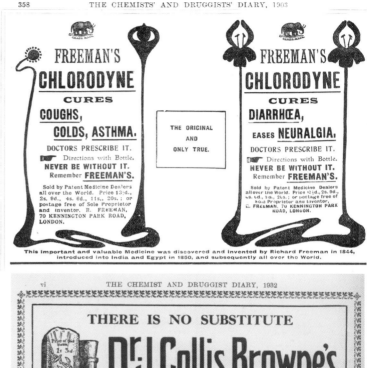

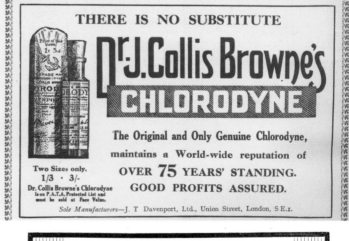

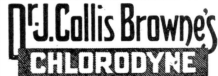

DR. J. COLLIS BROWNE'S

CHLORODYNE

Coughs, Colds, 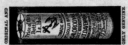 Asthma, Bronchitis,

Diarrhœa.

CHLORODYNE is admitted by the profession to be the MOST WONDERFUL AND VALUABLE REMEDY EVER DISCOVERED.

CHLORODYNE is the best remedy known for **COUGHS, COLDS, CONSUMPTION, BRONCHITIS, ASTHMA.**

CHLORODYNE effectually checks and arrests those too often fatal diseases: **DIPHTHERIA, FEVER, CROUP, AGUE.**

CHLORODYNE acts like a charm in **DIARRHŒA**, and is the only specific in **CHOLERA** and **DYSENTERY.**

CHLORODYNE effectually cuts short all attacks of **EPILEPSY, HYSTERIA, PALPITATION,** and **SPASMS.**

CHLORODYNE is the only palliative in **NEURALGIA, RHEUMATISM, GOUT, CANCER, TOOTHACHE,** and **MENINGITIS.**

The *Illustrated London News* of Sept. 28th, 1895, says :—

"If I were asked what single medicine I should prefer to take abroad with me, is likely to be most generally useful, to the exclusion of all others, I should say **CHLORODYNE.** I never travel without it, and its general applicability to the relief of a large number of simple ailments forms its best recommendation."

None genuine without the words "**DR. J. COLLIS BROWNE'S CHLORODYNE**" on the stamp. Overwhelming Medical testimony accompanies each bottle. Of all Chemists, 1/1½, 2/9, 4/6, & 11/-.

Sole Manufacturers : **J. T. DAVENPORT, Ltd., London.**

[TESTIMONIALS OTHER SIDE.]

Above and opposite: circa 1900 © private collection

❝ the most wonderful and valuable remedy ever discovered ❞

WONDERFUL AND VALUABLE REMEDY EVER DISCOVERED

CHLORODYNE Is the best remedy known for COUGHS, COLDS, CONSUMPTION, BRONCHITIS, ASTHMA

CHLORODYNE Effectually checks and arrests those too often fatal diseases; DIPHTHERIA, FEVER, CROUP, AGUE

CHLORODYNE Acts like a charm in DIARRHOEA, and is the only specific in CHOLERA and DYSENTERY

CHLORODYNE Effectually cuts short all attacks of EPILEPSY, HYSTERIA, PALPITATION, and SPASM

CHLORODYNE Is the only palliative in NEURALGIA, RHEUMATISM, GOUT, CANCER, TOOTHACHE, and MENINGITIS.

On the other side of the page are testimonials including:

Dr. GIBBONS, ARMY MEDICAL STAFF, CALCUTTA, states: "Two doses completely cured me of Diarrhoea."

ARCHBISHOP MAGEE.—Extract from one of his published letters to his wife:

"I had to return of a bad cold yesterday morning—preached with two pocket-handkerchiefs to a great congregation at St Mary's, ate a 'cold collation' at three o'clock, saw clergy on business until five o'clock, went to a 'parochial tea' at six o'clock; sat out no end of tea, glees, and speeches until half-past nine; finished off with a speech until ten o'clock, came here very bad with cold, took Chlorodyne and went to bed very miserable; woke next morning quite well."

From "CASSELL'S HISTORY OF THE BOER WAR," page 342:

"Gaunter and gaunter grew the soldiers of the Queen. Hunger and disease played havoc with those fine regiments. But somehow the R.A.M.C. managed to patch the men up with Chlorodyne and quinine."

EDWARD WHYMPER, Esq., the celebrated Mountaineer, writes on February 16th, 1897: — *"To J. T. DAVENPORT."*

"I always carry Dr. J. Collis Browne's Chlorodyne with me on my travels, and have used it effectively on others on Mont Blanc."

Martindale, 22nd edition 1943, quotes:

The medical properties of this remedy are anodyne, diaphoretic, sedative, astringent, antispasmodic. As a remedial agent in the treatment of febrile, inflammatory or neuralgic affections its administration has been found to exercise most remarkable curative effects in all stages of the disease.

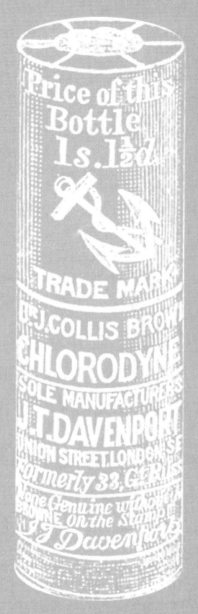

It is thought that the word Chlorodyne was derived from 'chloroform anodyne' as it contained chloroform and morphine. Although known to have been formulated by a qualified doctor, the Chlorodyne was regarded by some as a 'quack' medicine. In *Exposures of Quackery, Volume I*, the author complains that the product is dangerous, as a 1-ounce bottle (approximately 30 ml) contained 12 full doses of morphia and 36 full doses of chloroform. He continues:

the quantity of this and other chlorodynes sold is something enormous, far surpassing the imagination of anyone who has not given attention to the matter. Taken, at first, in small doses by the unhappy persons who drug themselves with chlorodyne, the victims become gradually habituated to its use and many fall, sooner or later, a prey to the craving for morphia. This craving once established, they become as completely slaves to the practice of swallowing chlorodyne in extraordinary quantities . . . with the inevitable consequence that physical, mental, and moral deterioration must follow.

Formula, 1874

Chloroform	4 ounces
Ether	1 ounce
Rectified spirit (alcohol)	4 ounces
Treacle	4 ounces
Extract of liquorice	2½ ounces
Muriate of morphia (hydrochloride)	8 grains
Oil of peppermint	16 minims
Syrup	17½ ounces
Prussic acid (2%)	2 ounces

Formula, 1872

Chloroform	6 drachms
Chloric ether	1 drachm
Tincture of capsicum	½ drachm
Oil of peppermint	2 minims
Hydrochlorate (hydrochloride) of morphia	8 grains
Hydrocyanic acid (Scheele's)	12 minims
Perchloric acid (hydrochloric acid)	20 grains
Tincture of Indian hemp	1 drachm
Treacle	1 drachm
	Dose: 5–10 drops

Formula, 1943

Liquid extract of opium (10% morphine)	1.4% w/v
Codeine	0.21% w/v
Chloroform	14% v/v
Proof spirit	5.75% v/v
Rectified tincture of capsicine	31% v/v
Peppermint oil	0.5% v/v
	Dose: 10–30 drops in a wineglassful of water

The formula was a secret. Peter Squire in his *Squire's Companion*, published from 1874, gave representational formula for 'those who object to *prescribe proprietary medicines*'. He named Chlorodyne LIQUOR CHLORO-FORMI COMPOSITUS.

Beasley, in 1872, published an additional formula from a Dr Ogden.

Squire's formula was adopted in the *British Pharmacopoeia*, 1885.

Martindale, 22nd edition 1943, gave the formula represented bottom left.

By 1969 the name had been changed to Collis Browne's Compound, codeine had been removed and the quantity of chloroform had been reduced.

In 1975 the President of the Pharmaceutical Society advised pharmacists that certain medicines should be subject to stronger controls owing to their abuse by the public and J Collis Browne's Compound was among them. It would be available only on prescription. The manufacturers discontinued the product and replaced it with a newly formulated preparation called J Collis Browne's Mixture.

In 1983, J Collis Browne's Tablets were introduced. The formulation of the mixture at the time of writing contains anhydrous morphine in peppermint water and the tablets contain light kaolin, morphine hydrochloride and calcium carbonate.

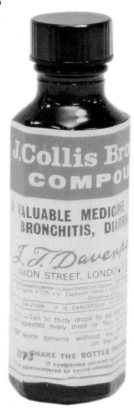

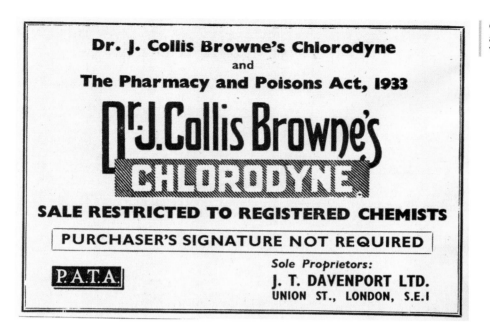

J Collis Browne's Chlorodyne was a medicine that worked. Its fault was that it relied heavily on, what are in today's world, substances of abuse. However, many people are still realising its benefits in the treatment of diarrhoea.

Formula, 1975

Opium liquid extract equivalent to morphine	1 mg
Peppermint oil	0.0015 ml
Capsicum tincture	0.0012 ml
Vehicle containing chloroform water	to 5 ml

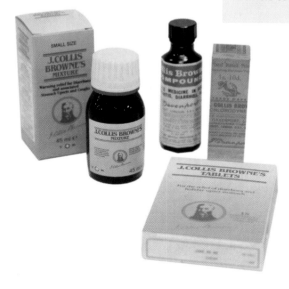

THE GENUINE IS

GELL'S DALBY'S   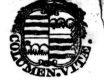   GELL'S DALBY'S

CARMINATIVE, CARMINATIVE,

WHICH, founded on just Medical Principles, is a most safe, effectual, and often, indeed, an immediate remedy, for the Wind, the Watery and Dry Gripes, Convulsions, and all those fatal Disorders in the Bowels of Infants which carry off such a number of the human species under the age of two years. It is also equally efficacious in *Gouty Pains* in the Intestines, in the *Bloody Flux*, and in the most *raking Colicks*, in GROWN PERSONS; and is particularly serviceable in those Fluxes and Disorders of the Bowels to which Seamen are subject.

It may not be improper to add that those Children who have been used to this Medicine are scarcely ever afflicted with *Worms*.

See over.

THE TRUE 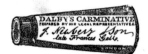 MEDICINE.

Can be procured through any Chemist in the civilized world, and at FRANCIS NEWBERY & SONS' WAREHOUSE, 1, KING EDWARD STREET, NEWGATE STREET, LONDON.

CAUTION.—WHEREAS many Counterfeited Preparations of this Medicine are sold by sundry Druggists and others, both at home and abroad, all Purchasers are requested to take notice that there is a seal (like the above) on the Cork of each Bottle; and that on the side of each Bottle is pasted a label, with these words—"*Dalby's Carminative, prepared by his legal representatives,*" and bearing the signature of "*F. Newbery & Sons.*" (See above representation.) Moreover, *in the Stamp* on each Bottle the name of "*F. Newbery,* No. 45, St. Paul's Churchyard," is engraved, which it would be a capital offence to imitate.

For the purpose of authentication, it may be well to observe that this Medicine was compounded by Mr. Anthony Gell (Coroner for Westminster), husband of Frances, daughter of the late Mr. Joseph Dalby, Apothecary, to whom only the secret was confided (see the extract from the will of Mr. Joseph Dalby, below), until his death in 1817, and from and after his death until the year 1858, by his son, Mr. John Henry Gell, of the Cloisters, Westminster Abbey (also Coroner for Westminster), and now by Mr. Robert Montague, his confidential assistant for many years before his death. Mr. Joseph Dalby in his life-time made arrangements by deed, dated 11th May, 1773, with Messrs. NEWBERY for the sale of this Medicine; these arrangements have never been disturbed. Purchasers of Dalby's Carminative should therefore be careful to ask for "Gell's," sold by Messrs. NEWBERY, and bearing their name.—*It is quite impossible that any other can be genuine.*

This Medicine is now prepared by the legal Representatives of Mrs. FRANCES GELL, Daughter of the late Mr. Joseph Dalby, Apothecary, the Inventor, to whom he bequeathed the same in the following words:—

EXTRACT FROM THE WILL OF MR. JOSEPH DALBY, PROVED A.D. 1784.

"*And Whereas I did many years since instruct my Daughter Frances, now the wife of Anthony Gell, of North Street, Westminster, Gentleman, in the art and method of preparing, compounding, and making up a certain Medicine, of which I am the sole Inventor, called and universally known by the name of DALBY'S CARMINATIVE; I have again instructed and communicated to my said Daughter, Frances Gell, the secret of preparing or making up the said Medicine; and I do hereby constitute and appoint my said Daughter the sole Preparer of this useful Medicine,—I likewise give to my said Daughter, Frances Gell, the sole Property of the said CARMINATIVE, and all Profits arising from the Sale thereof to Her or Her Heirs for ever.*"

DIRECTIONS FOR USING GELL'S DALBY'S CARMINATIVE.

First shake the Bottle until the contents are well mixed; and to a Child that is but two or three days old, and extremely weak, begin with 5 or 6 Drops; otherwise you may mix 10, 12, or 15 Drops of the Carminative in about a common spoonful (not more) of its food, made thin; or if the Child refuses its food, it should be given in warm water, sweetened with a little loaf sugar. If the dose should not give ease in six or eight minutes, repeat it, mixed as before; and as the Child grows older, increase the dose in proportion to its age and the violence of the symptoms.— Two Doses, or three at the most, in a day, will be sufficient, even in obstinate cases.

If a Dose were to be given once a day to all Children from two or three days to a fortnight or three weeks old, you might thereby prevent many Disorders to which the Bowels are liable, by carrying off that crude matter which frequently occasions them (the bad effects whereof are often manifested by Worms, Rickets, Ruptures, Convulsions, and other fatal symptoms), by strengthening the Stomach and Bowels, by causing good laudable chyle, and thereby establishing a good constitution.

In **Watery Gripes** or **Bloody Stools** you may repeat the Dose, proportioned to the age of the Patient, once in three or four hours, during the violence of the symptoms, afterwards every morning and evening till he recovers. To a Child from one to two years old, give a large Teaspoonful or more, if the symptoms are violent. To a Child of seven years old, three Teaspoonfuls. To a Grown Person, half or two-thirds of a Bottle at a Dose, either alone, or mixed with as much warm water as will make it lukewarm.

In **Gouty Pains** in the Stomach or Bowels, a Fit of the **Gravel** or **Colick** or in Painful **Flatulencies** of any kind, a Dose of the Carminative, properly proportioned according to these Directions, may be taken once in two or three hours, till the violence of the symptoms abates. In all very violent cases, a Grown Person should take a whole Bottle for the first Dose, and where an obstinate Costiveness prevails, and no stool is obtained by the Medicine, let a common Clyster be given, or a pint-and-a-half of Mutton Broth by way of Clyster, and repeated once in two hours till a stool is procured.

⁎⁎⁎ Till this is done, no effectual Relief will result from this or any other Medicine.

In curing the **Bloody Flux** this Medicine is very efficacious. In this case let the Patient, being fourteen years old and upwards, take half or two-thirds of a Bottle every morning and evening, or oftener, if the violence of the symptoms requires it.

⁎⁎⁎ Due regard should be had to the Patient's diet in all Colicks and all other Disorders of the Bowels.—Remember always to shake the Bottle well before you use it.

Sold Wholesale and Retail by F. NEWBERY and SONS, *at the only Warehouse for Dr. James's Fever Powder*, No. 1, King Edward Street, Newgate Street, London, E.C.; in Bottles, Price One Shilling and Ninepence each, duty included; and Purchasers are desired to observe that the words "F. NEWBERY, 45, St. Paul's Churchyard" (the old address of the Firm), are engraved in the Stamps, as the surest mark of authenticity, which they would do well to ascertain before they venture to take or administer the Carminative.

Sold also by the following Druggists; Sanger and Sons, *Oxford Street*; Sadler, *Norton Folgate*; Savory and Moore, *Bond Street*; Botwright and Kemp, *Islington*; Kemp, *Holloway*; Wright, *Kensington*; Tuck, *Mile End*; Atkins, *Woolwich*; Knight, *Wandsworth*; Moody, *Camberwell*; Howell, *Peckham*; Ragg, *Edmonton*; Bond, *Southgate*. Also in the following towns:—*Aberdeen*, Davidson; *Birmingham*, Arblaster; *Brighton*, Kemp and Glaisyer; *Bristol*, Ferris and Co.; *Beaumaris*, Slater; *Cranbrook*, Haselar; *Dover*, R. Wyles; *Hastings*, F. Rossiter; *Hoddesden*, Green; *Lincoln*, P. D. Woodcock; *Manchester*, Jewsbury and Brown; *Nottingham*, Smith and Co., G. Shepperly; *Norwich*, Corder; *Oxford*, Houghton and Son; *Preston*, Willan; *Plymouth*, Gibbons, Balkwill; *Ramsgate*, Fisher, Franks; *Reading*, Powell; *Ryde*, Gibbs and Gurnell; *Salisbury*, Brown; *Shrewsbury*, Blunt; *St. Leonard's*, Hempstead; *Tunbridge Wells*, Howard; *Windsor*, Russell; *York*, Raimes and Co.; and to be had of most Booksellers and Druggists throughout the Country.

THE CARMINATIVE SUFFERS NO INJURY BY KEEPING, OR BY CHANGE OF CLIMATE.

BE CAREFUL TO ASK FOR GELL'S DALBY'S CARMINATIVE.

Bearing on the Government Stamp the Name of "F. NEWBERY, 45, St. Paul's Churchyard," London.

See over.

Chapter Nine
Dalby's Carminative

alby's Carminative started life as a quack medicine and remained a popular remedy for stomach ailments for three centuries. It was thought to have been formulated by Joseph Dalby, son of an apothecary, Francis Dalby, who was a European émigré, possibly from France. Joseph Dalby owned an apothecary shop in Welbeck Street, London, and claimed that he first marketed his Carminative in 1773, but it may have been his father, Francis Dalby, who was the actual originator. Marketing was assigned to Francis Newbery and Sons, 45, St Paul's Churchyard, London.

Joseph Dalby died intestate in 1784 although he left an undated and unsigned will. In this will he wrote:

Whereas many years ago I taught my daughter Frances, now wife of Anthony Gell of North Street, Westminster, gent., to make my invented medicine called Dalby's Carminative . . . to preserve for the benefit of such of my children as deserve my attention and who have not by the most wanton indignities and unprovoked insolence forfeited all right and expectancy of any favour or kindness from me . . . I commend to my daughter Frances, the secret recipe.

Anthony Gell took over the business and added his own name to the product calling it Gell's Dalby's Carminative.

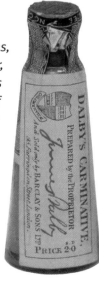
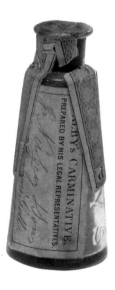

An undated flier in the collection of the Museum of the Royal Pharmaceutical Society continues the history:

For the purpose of authentication, it may be well to observe that this Medicine was compounded by Mr Anthony Gell (Coroner for Westminster), husband of Frances, daughter of the late Mr. Joseph Dalby, Apothecary, to whom only the secret was confided (see the extract from the will of Mr Joseph Dalby, below), until his death in 1817 and from and after his death until the year 1858, by his son, Mr John Henry Gell, of the Cloisters, Westminster Abbey (also Coroner for Westminster), and now by Mr Robert Montague, his confidential assistant for many years before his death.

(There then follows an embellished quotation of Joseph Dalby's unsigned will.)

To complicate matters, another Dalby's Carminative, manufactured by a James Dalby, was marketed through Barclay and Sons, 95 Fleet Market, London, from at least 1818. Another undated flier in the collection of the Museum of the Royal Pharmaceutical Society states:

CAUTION
To avoid spurious imitations care should be taken to refuse all preparations bearing any other name than JAMES DALBY.

As this medicine is prepared from the original recipe of the inventor, which has never left the possession of JAMES DALBY (his lineal descendant), it is a guarantee of its originality and purity.

The fliers from both products included similar logos which included the words 'COLUMEN VITAE' (the height of life).

Newbery and Sons continued to market Gell's Dalby's Carminative until 1934 and the James Dalby version was marketed by Barclay and Sons until 1939.

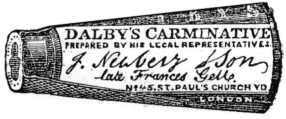

DALBY'S CARMINATIVE.

MADE IN COLUMEN VITÆ ENGLAND.

WHICH is founded on just medical principles, is a most safe, effectual, and often, indeed an immediate remedy for *Flatulence, Spasms, Diarrhœa*, and other disorders incidental to Infants. It is also equally efficacious in *Colics* in Grown Persons; and it is particularly serviceable in the disorders of the bowels to which seamen are subject. Children who have been used to this medicine are scarcely ever afflicted with flatulence.

NOTICE TO THE PURCHASER.

I, JAMES DALBY, of John's Row, in the parish of St. Luke's in the County of Middlesex, Gentleman, do hereby make oath, that having appointed Messrs. BARCLAY & SONS, 95, FLEET MARKET, LONDON, my sole and exclusive agents for the sale of the GENUINE DALBY'S CARMINATIVE; and in order that the said preparation may be rendered more secure from spurious Imitations, I have duly authorised them, from the date hereof, to affix the stamp containing their names and address to each bottle of the said medicine; and I do also make oath of the above Alteration in the putting up of the GENUINE DALBY'S CARMINATIVE prepared by me that the public may be duly guarded against all Counterfeits.

Sworn at the Mansion House, this 19th of December, 1818, before me JOHN ATKINS, Mayor.
JAMES DALBY, Proprietor.

DIRECTIONS FOR USING THE CARMINATIVE.

First shake the bottle until contents are well mixed; and to a child that is but two or three days old, begin with 5 or 6 drops, otherwise you may mix 10, 12 or 15 drops of the Carminative, in about a common spoonful, not more, of its food made thin; or if the child refuses its food, it should be given in warm water, sweetened with a little loaf sugar. If the dose does not give ease in 6 or 8 minutes, repeat it, mixed as before; and as the child grows older, increase the dose in proportion to its age and the violence of its symptoms. Two doses, or three at the most, in a day, will be sufficient even in obstinate cases.

In diarrhœa or dysentery you may repeat the dose, proportioned to the age of the patient, once in three or four hours, during the violence of the symptoms; afterwards every morning and evening until it recovers. To a child from one or two years old give a large tea-spoonful or more, if the symptoms are violent. To a child of seven years old, three tea-spoonfuls. To a grown person, half to two-thirds of a bottle at a dose; either alone or mixed with as much warm water as will make it lukewarm.

Children subject to costiveness or vomitings may take Fluid Magnesia with the Carminative to great advantage.

In a fit of the colic, or in flatulence of any kind, a dose of the Carminative, properly proportioned according to these directions, may be taken once in two or three hours, till the violence of the symptoms abates. In all very violent cases a grown person should take a whole bottle for the first dose; and where an obstinate costiveness prevails, and no stool is obtained by the medicine, let a common clyster be given, or a pint and a half of mutton broth by way of clyster, and repeated once in two hours until a stool is procured. Till this is done no effectual relief will result from this or any other medicine.

Due regard should be had to the patient's diet in all colics and other disorders of the bowels.—Remember always to shake the bottle well before you pour it out.

CAUTION!

To avoid spurious imitations care should be taken to refuse all preparations bearing any other name than JAMES DALBY.

As this medicine is prepared from the original recipe of the inventor, which has never left the possession of JAMES DALBY (his lineal descendant), it is a guarantee of its originality and purity. The public cannot be too particular to assure themselves that they really obtain JAMES DALBY'S Carminative, and that they are not imposed upon by any of the worthless imitations of this justly esteemed remedy, arising out of a celebrity sustained for upwards of 100 years. The genuine preparation is to be had only in bottles at 2/- each, properly stamped, sealed, and signed by JAMES DALBY, in red ink; and who, by way of affording the public a ready means of identifying it at first sight, has attached a band to the exterior of the wrapper containing the words—Prepared by JAMES DALBY, "the same as supplied to Her late Majesty's Troops in the Crimea, and to His Imperial Majesty the late Emperor of the French, etc.," and which he hopes will in some measure check the improper practices, pursued by unworthy medicine vendors, of occasionally substituting imitations of this the true and only genuine DALBY'S CARMINATIVE.

The Carminative suffers no injury by keeping or change of climate.

In all Export Orders to Foreign Countries, Printed Directions may be had in Hindustanee, French, German, Spanish, Dutch, Italian, Portuguese and other languages, if required.

EXCLUSIVE WHOLESALE AGENTS—BARCLAY & SONS, Limited, 95, Farringdon Street, London, E.C. 4.
SOLD BY ALL CHEMISTS, 2/- PER BOTTLE.
Hospitals, Infirmaries, Charitable Institutions, Exporters, and Public Departments liberally treated in contract supplies of large amount.

The following attestations among many others, of the success of the Carminative, have been sent to MR. DALBY.

"SIR,—About eighteen months since, I laboured under a complaint in my bowels in which I suffered the most excruciating pains for three months, and after having had medicines of two different gentlemen of the faculty, and could get no relief, I happily saw mention of your Carminative in a shop-bill of Mr. James Carey's, in Shepton Mallet. I sent for a bottle, which gave me immediate relief, and two more bottles nearly cured me, to the astonishment of all who knew my case; but going out too soon in the wet I contracted a cold, which brought on a relapse, so as to be nearly as bad as before. On sending for two bottles more, and taking half one, I obtained the usual relief, and the remainder completed the cure. "ROBERT PRINCE, Late of Allam, near Shepton Mallet, now of the Forest of Dean."

"Sir,—In August last (1892), at Paris during the progress of Asiatic Cholera, I had a severe attack of Cholerine, Dysentery, &c., and immediately had recourse to your Carminative, of which I always have a supply in store, knowing its efficiency both for Adults and Children. It is with unspeakable gratitude I inform you that one bottle restored me to my former health, and in justice to this valuable medicine I hereby return you many thanks." "EMILIE RAMEL, Rue Royer Collard, Paris."

"FIELD-MARSHAL LORD RAGLAN presents his compliments to the Proprietor of Dalby's Carminative, and begs to express to him his best thanks. He gratefully accepts the medicine for the relief and cure of Her Majesty's Troops suffering from Diarrhœa, etc." "Head Quarters before Sevastopol."

"THE INSPECTOR-GENERAL OF HOSPITALS, SIR JOHN HALL, in his report to Major-General Airey, the Quarter-Master General concerning the distribution of Dalby's Carminative placed at his disposal by the Field Marshall Commanding-in-Chief, when before Sevastopol, has stated that he also had occasion to take it himself, and that it afforded him almost immediate relief."

The Rev. GEORGE NICOL, of Kissy, Western Africa, to his friend, the Honourable J. T. COMMISSIONG, Collector of Customs and Member of the Council of Sierra Leone.

"MY DEAR SIR,—I must write to thank you for the Carminative, which safely arrived. It has done immense good, not only to the infant, but also to my little boy, now two years old. Accept my sincere thanks. The introduction of such a medicine will be of incalculable benefit to the Colony, and especially to Lagos and Abeokuta."

With kind regards, believe me, truly yours,
"Kissy Mission House, West Africa." GEORGE NICOL.

"SIR—I duly received the box of Carminative, and have reserved eleven bottles for the use of children, as I found it such a safe and effective remedy in the Bowel Complaints they are so frequently subject to. The medicine has been exceedingly useful, and the poor are extremely grateful; and from the Islands of St. Nicholas, St. Antonio, and St. Jago, to each of which I apportioned a store, I have received good accounts of the beneficial results. Believe me, yours very truly, THOMAS MILLER, H. M. Consul. "St. Vincent, Cape de Verde Islands."

The Gell's Dalby's Carminative was advertised as:

a most safe, effectual, and often, indeed an immediate remedy, for the Wind, the Watery and Dry Gripes, Convulsions, and all those fatal Disorders in the Bowels of Infants which carry off such a number of the human species under the age of two years. It is also equally efficacious in Gouty Pains in the Intestines, in the Bloody Flux, and in the most raking Colicks [sic], in Grown Persons; and is particularly serviceable in those Fluxes and Disorders of the Bowels to which Seamen are subject.

It may not be improper to add that those Children who have been used to this Medicine are scarcely ever afflicted with Worms.

James Dalby's claims were similar:

> ❝ Children who have been used to this medicine are scarcely ever afflicted with flatulence ❞

a most safe, effectual, and often, indeed an immediate remedy for Flatulence, Spasms and Diarrhoea, and other disorders incidental to Infants. It is also equally efficacious in Colics in Grown Persons; and is particularly serviceable in the disorders of the bowels to which seamen are subject. Children who have been used to this medicine are scarcely ever afflicted with flatulence.

The dosage of each product was very similar varying from five or six drops for an infant and up to two-thirds of a bottle for an adult. Both manufacturers made use of testimonials.

From Gell's:

Case of WILLIAM GAMLEN, Esq. at Zeal, near Tiverton, Devon.

"Being in great Disorder in my Bowels, and having tried several Medicines without Effect, I at last took Dalby's Carminative, which gave me immediate ease. Since that, a servant of mine was seized with a violent Flux and vomiting, which continued several

days, without relief; by taking one Bottle of the Medicine he was cured, and went to work the next day.

> *WILLIAM GAMLEN*

And from James Dalby's:

FIELD-MARSHALL LORD RAGLAN presents his compliments to the Proprietor of Dalby's Carminative, and he begs to express to him his best thanks. He gratefully accepts the medicine for the relief and cure of Her Majesty's Troops suffering from diarrhoea, etc.

Head Quarters before Sevastopol [sic].

Gray's Supplement, 1848, gave a formula (see below).

These appear to be the ingredients always used for the James Dalby/Barclay's version. The same formula is given in *Martindale*, 21st edition.

The contents given in *The Lancet*, 28 November 1903 were powdered rhubarb, magnesium carbonate, glycerine, sugar, peppermint oil, dill oil and a small quantity of laudanum (tincture of opium).

The reason that Dalby's Carminative was available for almost 170 years was undoubtedly its efficacy. The ingredients were well tried and tested and very suitable for indigestion and diarrhoea. Similar prescribable medicines included Aromatic Mixture of Magnesium Carbonate Compound, B.P. 2003, which contained magnesium carbonate and aromatic oils.

Formula, 1848

Carbonate of magnesia	2 drachms
Oil of peppermint	1 minim
Oil of nutmegs	2 minims
Oil of aniseed	3 minims
Tincture of castor	30 minims
Tincture of assafoetida	10 minims
Tincture of opium	5 minims
Spirit of pennyroyal	15 minims
Compound tincture of cardamoms	30 minims
Peppermint water	2 fluid ounces

Fennings'

CHILDREN'S COOLING POWDER'S

FOR CHILDREN CUTTING THEIR TEETH

SOLD IN BOXES 1'3, 3'- 1d OR 2 FOR 1½d.

Chapter Ten

*F*ennings' Children's Cooling Powders

*I*f you walk out of London Bridge station and cross Tooley Street towards the river Thames, you are confronted by a large office block, the headquarters of the management consultancy company PricewaterhouseCoopers, and next to it, a shopping complex called Hay's Galleria. Until the 1960s, this area was part of the thriving London docks. Hay's Galleria, previously Hay's Wharf, began its life as Fennings' Wharf, and was founded by Mr Fennings in 1832. Although the wharf was totally destroyed by fire in 1849, it was completely rebuilt and continued to develop. Today, the only surviving clue to the Fennings family's links to the area is a Fennings Street.

Mr Fennings the wharfinger had a son called Alfred, and this is where the pharmaceutical story begins. Dr Alfred Fennings, now a graduate of Edinburgh University, opened the Golden Key Pharmacy at Hammersmith Broadway in 1840. Records show him renting a house and yard on the Broadway at a rent of £27 per annum until the spring of 1851. Fennings surfaces in the records again on 9 December 1851 when he married Angelina Steinberg, one of his landladies in Hammersmith, in the parish church of Northwood in Cowes, Isle of Wight. On the marriage certificate he is described as 'batchelor and

Fennings' CHILDREN'S Cooling POWDERS
FOR CHILDREN CUTTING THEIR TEETH FOR MILD FEVERISH CONDITIONS AND GENERAL RESTLESSNESS AND FOR PAIN ARISING FROM SWOLLEN GUMS, THRUSH, ETC.
When necessary ONE DOSE may be given in the evening in a little water, or placed dry into the open mouth, the baby's head being held back gently for a few seconds.
20 POWDERS · 20 POWDERS

Physician' and she as 'spinster'. Her father was described as a merchant. Angelina was nine years older than Fennings.

Dr Fennings' move to Cowes on the Isle of Wight was a very fashionable one. Queen Victoria's summer home, Osborne House, just outside Cowes, was finished in 1851. Meanwhile, Fennings opened a small factory to make his own formulas on the island. From the beginning of his time on the Isle of Wight, Fennings advertised that he would send remedies directly by post from Cowes if requested by a customer.

Fennings specialised in treatments for cholera, typhus and other fevers. Preparations available in the early days were Fennings' Fever Curer [sic] and Fennings' Stomachic Mixture for the treatment of cholera, fevers and flu. Fennings' Cooling Powders were produced for teething problems and Fennings' Lung Healers, later called Little Healers, were developed for the treatment of coughs and colds. Fennings claimed that his Fever Curer could cure bowel complaints with one dose, diphtheria with three doses, cholera with five and influenza with six.

Fennings also wrote many pamphlets and articles on the treatment of cholera and on child welfare in general, including 'On the Cause and Cure of Bronchitis, Cause and Cure of Typhus Fever, Volcanic Origins of Cholera, and Whooping Cough and its Remedy'.

He died on 7 January 1900, aged 85. The profits from his business clearly meant that he had been able to live a comfortable life. A note in The Chemist and Druggist, 1901 stated:

> At Cowes last week a quantity of the personal effects of the late Mr Alfred Fennings, the well-known Cowes patent-medicine proprietor, was brought under the hammer. There were no fewer than thirty-six pairs of gentlemen's fancy-worked slippers, scarcely any of which had ever been worn, and a large number of black suits of clothes, perfectly new.

Fennings left his business to be administered by his trustees, WJ Bailey, HB Wallen and FB Pelly. He instructed that his business should be continued and that all profits should be devoted to a national children's charity. From 1900 to 1984, over £2 million had been donated to charity. During his lifetime, Fennings also contributed regularly to the Pharmaceutical Society's Benevolent Fund.

The first insight into the formulas of Fennings' products came in *Secret Remedies*. Each dose of Fennings' Children's Cooling Powders, with an average weight of 3.4 grains (0.22 g), contained potassium chlorate 70% and powdered liquorice 30%. The estimated cost of these ingredients in a 2/9d box (about 14p) was one-sixth of a penny. Each Fennings' Lung-Healers pill only contained ipecachuana and an excipient used to bind the powder into pills. The estimated cost of the ingredients for 30 pills (sold for 1/1½d) was a halfpenny. In 1984, Fennings promoted the fact that the formula for this product, then called Little Healers, had been unchanged for 137 years, with 15 million tablets sold annually, mainly in Lancashire, which was the home of the main distribution depot. Fennings sold 17 million Little Healers in a month during the Asian flu epidemic in 1957 – 1958.

In volume 2 of *Exposures of Quackery*, written by the anonymous editor of *Health News* in 1895, analysis of the Fever Curer sought to test the claim that Fennings' product could cure yellow fever, typhus fever, cholera and small pox:

> *In his gamut of the curative properties of the Fever Curer, he carries up to what six doses will do. If seven would only cure lying, what a boon it would be in his case . . .*

The analysis showed that it was a dilute solution of nitric acid, flavoured with peppermint and containing minute traces of other organic matter, including a very small amount of opium. The analyst, Professor Wanklyn, noted that the bottle's wrapper was marked poison, and the need for this was explained because it contained a few drops of laudanum, described as a '*most beneficial physic*'. However, he noted that there was not enough in the remedy to be described in this way: '*as barefaced a falsehood as the assertion that Fennings' Fever Curer has for nearly fifty years been curing thousands of cases of diseases which "no other medicine could cure"*'. Wanklyn was also critical of the dose being specified as a wineglass because these vary in size.

Formula, 1943

Potassium chlorate	30%
Liquorice	33%
Powdered malt	33%
Light magnesium carbonate	4%

Formula, 1955

Bromvaleton	10%
Calcium phosphate	28%
Lactose	14%
Liquorice	33%
Phenacetin	10%
Heavy magnesium oxide	5%

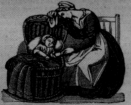

EVERY MOTHER'S BOOK;

OR,

The Child's Best Doctor.

BY

ALFRED FENNINGS,

AUTHOR OF TREATISES "ON THE CAUSE AND CURE OF BRONCHITIS," "CAUSE AND CURE
OF TYPHUS FEVER," "VOLCANIC ORIGIN OF CHOLERA," "HOOPING
COUGH AND ITS REMEDY," ETC.

CONTAINING THE BEST MEANS TO CURE

Coughs		Looseness
Colds		Worms, &c.
Convulsions		Measles
Chicken Pox		Mumps
Eruptions		Nettle Rash
Fevers		Red Gum
Gripes		Rashes
Hooping Cough		Ringworm

Sores	Scarlet Fever	Thrush
Sore Eyes	Scarlatina	Wind
Sore Throats	Scald Head	Weaning Brash
Sore Nipples	Teething	Watery Brain

The OMNISCIENT GOD never intended that nearly half of the babies born in
this country should die, as they now do, before they are five years of age. Carelessness, poisonous white Calomel Powders, and a general ignorance of simple safe remedies
to cure their peculiar diseases, have been the fatal causes.

ENTERED AT STATIONERS' HALL.

The formula for Fennings' Children's Cooling Powders changed over time. In 1943, the medicine consisted of potassium chlorate, liquorice, powdered malt and light magnesium carbonate. By 1955, phenacetin, bromvaleton and calcium phosphate featured.

In the 25th edition of *Martindale*, published in 1967, the bromvaleton, a hypnotic, had been removed. By the following edition, published in 1972, the phenacetin, an antipyretic and analgesic, had been replaced with paracetamol. By 2005, the Cooling Powders were the only Fennings preparation still available, and the only active ingredient in them was paracetamol.

Fennings' advertising did not pull any punches. A 1901 advert in *The Chemists' and Druggists' Diary* was headed '*Do not let your child die!*' and '*Do not untimely die*'. One of Fennings' primary channels for advertising was free booklets that were issued through pharmacies or directly by post. The two titles were *Everybody's Doctor* and *Every Mother's Book*. The melodramatic tone of the advertising continued in the booklets. Fennings' Fever Curer was advocated:

A Bottle should be kept in every House, to be ready for use day or night. In some Diseases, an hour's delay is a life lost. Have a Remedy always ready at hand.

The preface of *Every Mother's Book* dated 1857 stated:

The theme [of the booklet] *shall still be the necessity of yourself becoming your Child's only Doctor—and its object, the safety of the little earth-angel that nestles in your bosom, and the life-preservation of the small loved ones who lisp you Mother.*

The preface goes on to ask the mother to make three resolutions: to use her reason that enables her to understand difficult crochet patterns to understanding basic medical facts, not to use mineral powders, and to use simply harmless physic, and definitely not leeches or the lancet to bleed her children.

Fennings continued to promote their Children's Cooling Powders as free from dangerous chemicals. They stated on the packaging '*Do not contain calomel, opium, morphia, nor anything injurious to a tender babe*'. The advice was that the powders could be given mixed with water, or thrown dry into the opened mouth of the baby. The mother should then gently hold back its head for half a minute until it swallows it. *Every Mother's Book* (1857) warned against '*the present Medical mania for prescribing Mineral Poisons and Deadly Drugs*', and another stated '*The OMNISCIENT GOD never intended that nearly half of the Babies born in this country should die, as they now do, before they are five years of age. Carelessness, poisonous white Calomel Powders, and a general ignorance of simple safe remedies, to cure their peculiar diseases, have been the fatal causes.*'

Later editions of *Every Mother's Book* covered a range of issues relating to bringing up a new baby including advice on sleep patterns to rest a baby's 'tiny brain', fresh air, feeding, washing, teething and the full gamut of childhood diseases that could be treated using Fennings' products. The booklet intersperses adverts and directions for using these products with 'General Hints'. The 1934 edition begins:

Every baby to-day is born into a world of opportunities undreamed of a generation

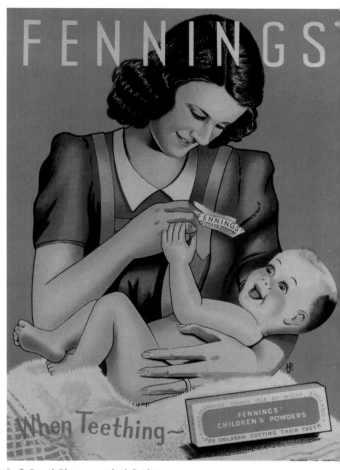

© Royal Pharmaceutical Society

> **Do not contain calomel, opium, morphia, nor anything injurious to a tender babe**

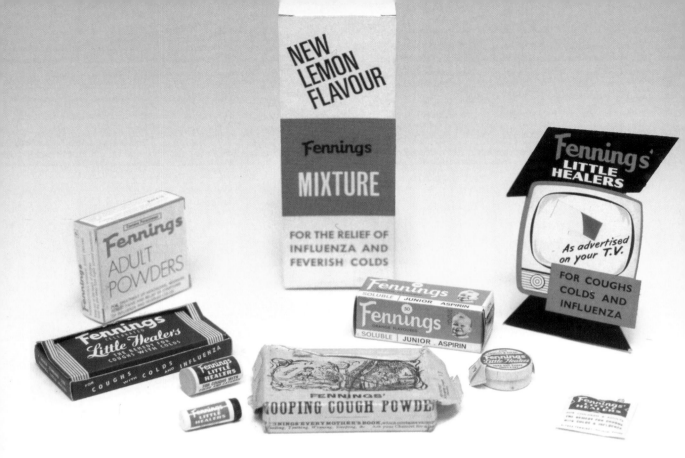

ago . . . This little book is intended to guide and help mothers faced with the responsibility of bringing a child through its early critical years, which affect, for good or ill, its health throughout the whole of the rest of its life . . . A number of remedies are here recommended for children's illnesses. They are safe and simple remedies which mothers have used for over seventy years. Pleasant in use and easy to administer, they contain nothing which might injure the delicate constitution of a baby.

An advert in 1931 shows that the Fennings' product range consisted of Children's Powders, Adult Powders, Lung Healers, Stomach Strengtheners, Fever Curer, Hooping [sic] Cough Powders, Worm Powders and Rheumatic Drops. Fennings moved from Cowes to Horsham, West Sussex, in 1950, although most of the manufacturing took place in Mabelthorpe, Lincolnshire, and the main distribution depot was in Ashton-under-Lyne in Lancashire. The company changed name from Alfred Fennings to Fennings Pharmaceuticals in 1969. A promotional booklet from around this date described the fever mixture as a '*famous Preparation for arresting the symptoms of influenza and one which should be kept in every family medicine ches*t'. The adult cooling powders seem to have been promoted as a hangover cure: '*These powders are excellent for cooling mild feverishness, for the relief of headache and for dispersing that "early morning" feeling*'. Other products in this booklet include rheumatic tablets, cough mixture, ointment, tablets for heartburn, and antiseptic baby powder containing hexachlorophene. An additional advert, again from this period, promotes Fennings' Ointment for:

> *abrasions, abscesses, aching feet, blotches, bruises, burns, boils, chapped hands, chilblains, cuts, eczema, erythema, festering sores, heat rashes, insect bites, inflammation, nettlerash, psoriasis, scalds, sprains, stings, sunburn, ulcers, poisoned wounds etc.*

The product range was therefore large. It seems to have expanded again in 1984 to include soluble junior aspirin, gripe mixture, specially formulated children's shampoo, and four formulations for adults – to relieve the symptoms of feverish colds, flu, irritating coughs and stomach upsets. In 1989, Fennings' products began to be distributed by Waterhouse. The range contracted to simply Adult and Children's Cooling Powders, Gripe Mixture, Little Healers, and Lemon Flavour Mixture for Influenza. Waterhouse took over completely in 1994 when the product range dropped the Adult Cooling Powders. In 1998, Fennings' products, then just Children's Cooling Powders and Little Healers, were taken over by Anglian Pharma, based in Hertfordshire.

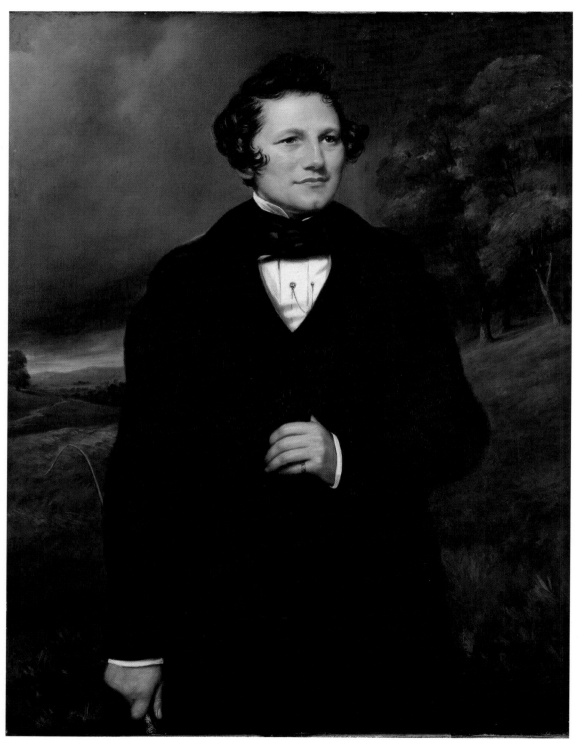

Chapter Eleven
*H*olloway's Pills and Ointment

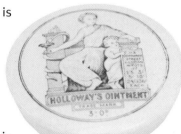

*T*he story of Holloway's Pills and Ointment is another based on the power of advertising. They were quack remedies but their formulas produced effects that could be identified by people who succumbed to the tremendous impact of marketing.

Thomas Holloway was born on 22 September 1800 in an inn called the 'Robin Hood and Little John' in Devonport (then called Plymouth Dock), Devon. His father ran a bakery and a number of inns in the area. The Holloway family moved a number of times, arriving at the 'Turk's Head' in Penzance in about 1811. Following the death of his father, he shared a grocery shop in the market place with his mother and his brother.

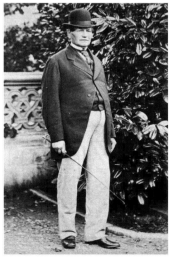

In 1828, Holloway moved to Roubaix, France. On his return he had various jobs including that of an interpreter. In 1836 he opened a business in Broad Street, London, as a merchant and foreign commercial agent. It was during this time that he commenced making his ointment and pills. It has been said that he received a formula for an ointment from Felix Albinolo from Turin, a leech seller who wanted to market his own ointment. Holloway helped him

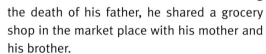

RHC PH 281/4/1. Archives, Royal Holloway, University of London

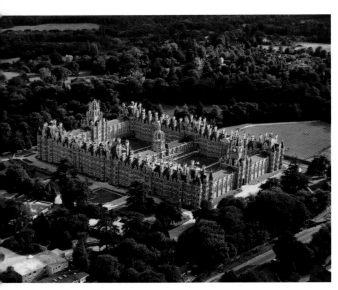

by introducing him to the authorities at St Thomas' Hospital as the inventor of a new ointment but the hospital was not prepared to endorse the product. Holloway decided that it might be worth while making and promoting a similar product to the general public and in 1837 launched Holloway's Family Ointment.

In 1840, Holloway married Miss Jane Driver and she helped him by working long hours to prepare his pills and ointment. He added the title Professor to his name as a commercial ploy but abandoned the title in later life. His main method to promote his wares was to visit Plymouth Dock where he would make captains, crews and passengers of ships travelling to all parts of the world, aware of his products. He then tried advertising in local papers.

In his own words:

It was on the 15th October, 1857, that my first Advertisement appeared. The Medicines were not offered unto the public, or indeed known to them until that period.

My beginning was in a small way—my task very difficult and quite disheartening.

I may add as a proof of my early discouragement that I had expended in one week the sum of £500 in various other ways for the purpose of my business, and I only sold in that time two small pots of ointment. In fact, no person would then have accepted the Medicines as a gift.

HOLLOWAY'S PILLS AND OINTMENT

Have the Largest Sale of any Medicine in the World.

MANUFACTURED ONLY AT

Professor HOLLOWAY'S Establishment,

78 New Oxford St. (late 533 Oxford St.), London.

And sold at 1s. 1½d., 2s. 9d., 4s. 6d., 11s., 22s., *and* 33s. *each Box or Pot.*

Chemists and Druggists selling "Holloway's Pills and Ointment" can, on application to the above address, or to the Wholesale House with whom they deal, be supplied free of charge with Handbills and Posters with their name and address printed at foot.

For Wholesale Terms see List of "Proprietary Articles" in most Price Currents.

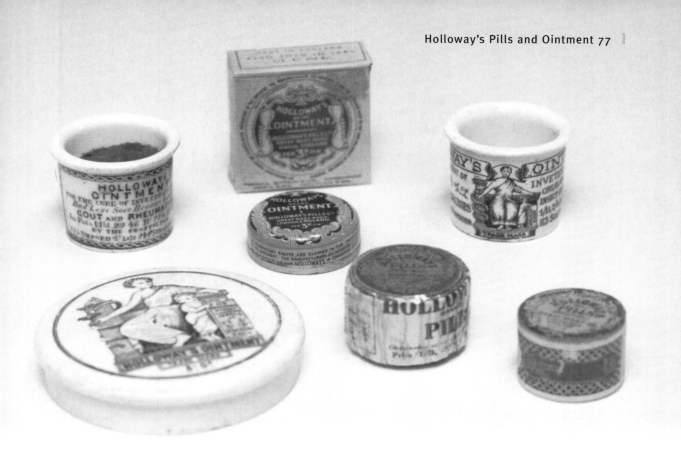

I had to practice the most rigid economy and also to work most assiduously. By 4 o'clock in the morning I had generally commenced my day not to cease until 10 at night in order to do that for myself for which else I may have paid others.

It was rumoured that one of his promotional methods was to send his brother Henry into selected shops to ask for Holloway's famous pills and ointment, and then to pretend amazement that they were not stocked. Later in the day Thomas Holloway would enter the store as an agent for his own remedies and secure orders.

Unfortunately Holloway grossly overspent on advertising and ran into debt. He was committed to the debtor's prison in Whitecross Street, London. On release, he moved to the Strand, near Temple Bar, where he resumed trading. The 1839 *London Directory* entry states 'Thomas Holloway, Patent Medicine Warehouse, 244 Strand'. He started advertising again in a smaller, more selective way. When his mother died in 1843 it was discovered that she had advanced him £600 that was never

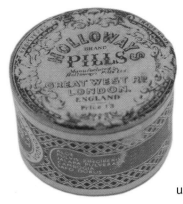

repaid. By 1864 the size of his premises had increased and his volume of sales exceeded £250,000 per annum. In 1867 the premises were compulsorily purchased by the Law Courts and Holloway moved to 533 New Oxford Street which he named Holloway House.

His advertising spread all over the world and his products sold well in all countries except France. To use his own words again:

It was a rule with me from commencement to spend judiciously all the money I could spare in publicity which went on increasing, and in the year 1842 I expended about £5000 in advertising.

Time rolled on, and from the hitherto unthought of yearly outlay of £5000 I increased it to £10,000 in the year 1845. At the time of the Great Exhibition in London in 1851 my expenditure was £20,000 per annum; in the year 1855 the Cost of publicity had risen to the sum of £30,000; and in the present year (1864) it has reached £40,000 in advertising my medicines in every available manner throughout this globe.

For the proper application of their use I have had the most ample directions translated into every known tongue—such as Chinese, Turkish, Armenian, Arabic, Sanskrit and most of the vernaculars of India, and all the languages spoken on the European Continent.

He boasted:

Among my Correspondents I number Kings and Princes, equally with other distinguished foreigners, of all Nations. When the Ambassadors from Siam visited London in 1857, they were not only the bearer to me of an Autograph letter from their Major Hing, but also of a gold enameled ornament which they delivered here, arriving in one of the Queen's private carriages with a Prince Interpreter, who informed me, on the feast of the Ambassadors that this honour was paid to me as a testimony of His Majesty's satisfaction on learning that my remedies were introduced into his dominions, and with marked benefit to many of his subjects.

The Ambassadors ordered at the same time, for His Majesty's use, Five pounds worth of my pills and ointment, which were sent to their Hotel (Claridges) Brook Street, Grosvenor Square.

'His Majesty' was King Monkut of Siam – of *The King and I* musical fame.

Holloway possessed such commercial strength that one of his conditions of using a paper or periodical was that he should receive a copy bearing his advertisement so that it could be carefully scrutinised. In this way he built up one of the largest collections in the world of English, colonial and foreign newspapers and periodicals.

Holloway died on 26 December 1883. The business continued under the management of his nephew Sir George Martin Holloway. In 1929 the business was incorporated as a limited liability company, Holloways Pills Ltd, and in 1931 was acquired by Beechams Pills Ltd, which then acquired the rights to the licences for 'Holloway's Pills' and Holloway's Ointments. The pills were manufactured at the former factory of

Reproduced with permission from *The Chemists' and Druggists' Diary*, 1903

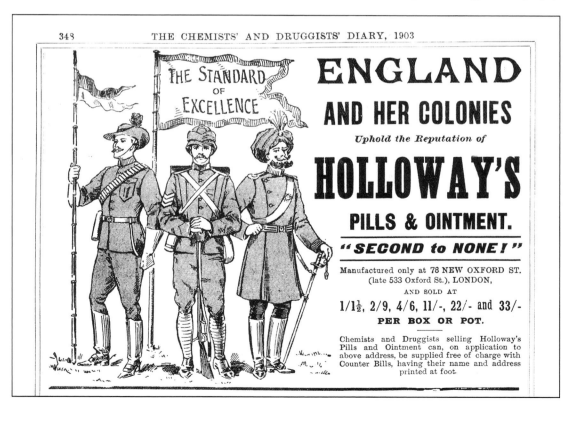

348   THE CHEMISTS' AND DRUGGISTS' DIARY, 1903

THE STANDARD OF EXCELLENCE

ENGLAND AND HER COLONIES

Uphold the Reputation of

HOLLOWAY'S PILLS & OINTMENT.

" SECOND to NONE ! "

Manufactured only at 78 NEW OXFORD ST. (late 533 Oxford St.), LONDON,

AND SOLD AT

1/1½, 2/9, 4/6, 11/-, 22/- and 33/-

PER BOX OR POT.

Chemists and Druggists selling Holloway's Pills and Ointment can, on application to above address, be supplied free of charge with Counter Bills, having their name and address printed at foot.

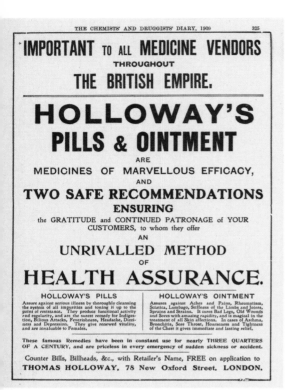

THE CHEMISTS' AND DRUGGISTS' DIARY, 1909   325

IMPORTANT TO ALL MEDICINE VENDORS
THROUGHOUT
THE BRITISH EMPIRE.

HOLLOWAY'S
PILLS & OINTMENT
ARE
MEDICINES OF MARVELLOUS EFFICACY,
AND
TWO SAFE RECOMMENDATIONS
ENSURING
the GRATITUDE and CONTINUED PATRONAGE of YOUR
CUSTOMERS, to whom they offer
AN
UNRIVALLED METHOD
OF
HEALTH ASSURANCE.

HOLLOWAY'S PILLS | **HOLLOWAY'S OINTMENT**

Assure against serious illness by thoroughly cleansing the system of all impurities and toning it up to the point of resistance. They produce functional activity and regularity, and are the surest remedy for Indigestion, Bilious Attacks, Feverishness, Headache, Dizziness and Depression. They give renewed vitality, and are invaluable to Females.

Assures against Aches and Pains, Rheumatism, Sciatica, Lumbago, Stiffness of the Limbs and Joints, Sprains and Strains. It cures Bad Legs, Old Wounds and Sores with amazing rapidity, and is magical in the treatment of all Skin affections. In cases of Asthma, Bronchitis, Sore Throat, Hoarseness and Tightness of the Chest it gives immediate and lasting relief.

These famous Remedies have been in constant use for nearly THREE QUARTERS OF A CENTURY, and are priceless in every emergency of sudden sickness or accident.

Counter Bills, Billheads, &c., with Retailer's Name, FREE on application to
THOMAS HOLLOWAY, 78 New Oxford Street, LONDON.

Reproduced with permission from *The Chemists' and Druggists' Diary*, 1907

Holloways Pills Ltd at Clipstone Street, London, and the ointment was made by Veno Drug Co Ltd at the same factory. Production ceased in 1951.

Thomas Holloway was a great benefactor. He was not interested in charities because he felt that they *'demeaned the poor'* but he did believe in benevolence. He was very interested in insanity in the middle and upper classes of society. The price of treatment in institutions for the upper classes of society was prohibitive to the middle classes although asylums for the poor were plentiful. In 1864 Holloway decided that he would build a sanatorium directed to the middle classes. His wife laid the first stone, he laid the second and the landscape gardener the third. He wrote:

I have erected, at a cost of £200,000 a Sanatorium for the cure of mental disorders, and endowed it with £50,000. It is situated within two miles of Egham and near to Virginia Water Station. It will accommodate 125 males, and the same number of females of the middle Class. It will be nearly self-supporting. Neither epileptic, paralytic or presumed incurable patients can be received. Patients cannot remain for a longer period than twelve months and no patient can be readmitted.

The building, named 'The Holloway Sanatorium', still stands on raised ground near Virginia Water Station. It is constructed of red brick, with some Portland stone dressings, and is in the Gothic style, the particular treatment shown on the exterior being continued in the internal decorations.

In 1873 Mrs Holloway died. Holloway turned his energy to building a ladies' college near Egham in Surrey, not far from the sanatorium. This is the Royal Holloway College which he dedicated to the memory of his wife. He wrote:

I have deemed it my duty to make some acknowledgements to the public for the means which through them I possess. In furtherance of this intention I have commenced the building of a College for Women of the middle and upper middle Classes on an estate of ninety five acres, situated within one mile of Egham, and 18 miles of London. It will have a capacity to accommodate 250 students with two private rooms for each. A duly qualified Lady Physician will reside in the College.

The curriculum of the College will be in some measure similar to that of the Universities of Oxford and Cambridge. I shall provide for the foundation of twenty scholarships of forty pounds each.

It will not be a training College for Teachers and Governesses. The terms for residence will be the same for all students. The building with its furniture is estimated to cost about £250,000, to which I shall add an endowment of £100,000.

The College with its associations and teaching will, I hope be acceptable to the public of this Country and its dependencies.

Royal Holloway, University of London, was formed in 1985 by the amalgamation of Royal Holloway and Bedford Colleges, both originally women's colleges of the University of London, which admitted male undergraduates in 1965.

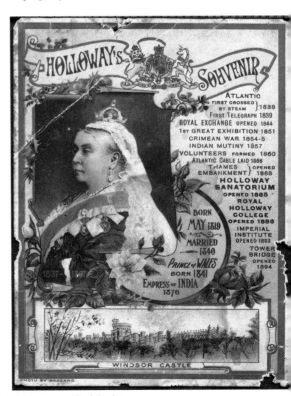

Holloway did not live to see the opening of either of his buildings. The sanatorium was opened on 15 June 1885 by the Prince of Wales and the college by Queen Victoria on 30 June 1886.

A flier from the collection of the Museum of the Royal Pharmaceutical Society offers a testimonial from Mr James McKenna, Royal Oak Farm, Santry, near Dublin dated 29 May 1866.

PROFESSOR HOLLOWAY

Sir—Two years ago I lost the use of my limbs—they were quite benumbed; my sight was becoming numbed, my hearing dull, and pains which had plagued me for twenty years, were growing worse. I consulted the most eminent of the faculty without deriving any benefit. About a month since I was induced to try your Pills and Ointment, and I feel myself in duty bound to make known to you and the public the miraculous change they wrought in me in a few days. On the fourth day I perceived a change for the better; my pulse began to beat stronger the blood to circulate more freely than it had flown for years, my sight to receive its former clearness, and my hearing to be as acute as ever. I am now, thanks to God and your invaluable Pills and Ointment, quite recovered, and am able to follow my usual avocations with comfort.

I remain, yours gratefully,
JAMES MCKENNA

> **A Key to Health!!! The Hollowayian System of Medicine and its adaptation for the treatment of many Diseases incident to the human frame**

Holloway's Pills were featured in *More Secret Remedies*. It quotes from a pamphlet round the box entitled '*A Key to Health!!! The Hollowayian System of Medicine and its adaptation for the treatment of many Diseases incident to the human frame*'. It goes on to state that the 'Hollowayian System' meant taking the pills and applying the ointment simultaneously. This would treat gout, rheumatism, sciatica, paralysis, liver complaints, asthma, inflammation of the kidneys, bronchitis, quinsy, bad legs, bad breasts, ulcers wounds, sores, tumours, piles and fistulas, the turn of life, floodings and the whites, obstruction of the menses, dropsies, jaundice, youthful indiscretion, impotency, palpitation of the heart, debility, indigestion, constipation, gravel, stone, venereal diseases, influenza. Erysipelas, lepra blotches, scald heads and ringworms, scrofula, ague, diarrhoea, etc.

The dose varied from two pills a day to seven pills night and morning.

Chemical and microscopical examination showed that the ingredients were aloes, powdered ginger and soap – at best a laxative action. *Secret Remedies* did not analyse the ointment.

In *Exposures of Quackery*, volume I, 1895, the results of analysis by a 'Mons. Dorvault, an eminent French chemist' gave the formulas for the pills and ointment.

The Extra Pharmacopoeia 1943 states:

Holloway's Brand Ointment *'For the treatment of ulcers, cuts, chilblains, chapped hands, wounds, burns, bruises, insect bites, boils, bad legs, etc.'* Formula:—Cera Flav. (yellow beeswax) 19.2%, Tereb. Venet. Fact (Venetian turpentine) 28.80%, Butter Fat 52.00%.

Holloway's Brand Pill *'Act by purifying the system, regulating the functions, harmonising the bodily workings, enriching and cleansing the blood, toning liver, kidneys and excretory organs, ensuring full nourishment from your food, strengthening the whole body.'* Formula:—Aloe 36.15%, Pulvis Zingiberis (powdered ginger) 36.15%, Jalap Pulverata (powdered jalap) 12.00%, Cambogia 12.00%, Sapo Dura (hard soap) 3.70%. Dose 2 to 6 pills.

Thomas Holloway was a very rich man, some say a millionaire. Fortunately, he wished to preserve his name and this he has done through his architectural creations. He was, in his own time, criticised for his hard-hitting advertising. In *Exposures of Quackery*, volume I, 1895, the following anecdote was printed:

When Charles Dickens was in the height of his splendid career as a novelist, Holloway sent him a cheque for £1000, with an intimation that he might consider it as his property if he would insert in an early number of one of his works, then coming out in a serial form, some reference to the Holloway patent medicines. Dickens, to his honour be it said, with equal promptitude and indignation, returned the proffered bribe. Upon hearing of this incident, Thackeray remarked, with the quiet sarcasm of which he was the master, that if he had been in Dickens' place he would have killed the villain of the novel with an overdose of Holloway's Pills, and thus have secured the £1000.

Punch described Holloway and Morison 'as *the most remarkable PILLERS of society*'.

Formula, 1895

In 144 pills:	
Aloes	62 grains
Rhubarb	27 grains
Saffron	3 grains
Sulphate of soda	3 grains
Pepper	3 grains

Formula, 1895

The ointment:	
Olive oil	$62\frac{1}{2}$ parts
Lard	50 parts
Resin	25 parts
White wax	$12\frac{1}{2}$ parts
Yellow wax	3 parts
Turpentine	3 parts
Spermaceti	3 parts

"The Three Doctors"

Dr. Francis Newbery being introduced by Dr. Saml. Johnson to Dr. Robt. James 1767

With Hearty Greetings and Best Wishes
for a
Prosperous New Year
from
FRANCIS R. L. NEWBERY
F.R.S.A.

Francis Newbery (Charterhouse) Ltd.

to his many friends
At Home and Abroad

18-21, CHARTERHOUSE SQUARE,
LONDON, E.C.I, ENGLAND.

Clerkenwell 5338
6392
6393

Cablegrams
Radiograms } NEWBERY
Telegrams   LONDON.

Chapter Twelve
Dr James's Fever Powder

The history of Dr James's Fever Powder has been dominated by the attempts of others to establish its formula and the method by which it was made.

Dr Robert James, the son of an army officer, was born in 1705 at Kinvaston in Staffordshire and went to school at Lichfield Grammar. His classmate, Samuel Johnson, remained a lifelong friend. James went to St John's College, Oxford, where he obtained a BA degree in 1726. In 1728 he became an extra licentiate of the College of Physicians of London. James practised in Lichfield, Sheffield, Birmingham, and finally London. He first lived at Southampton Street, Covent Garden, and then Craven Street, off the Strand.

James's Powder was patented by Dr James on 13 November 1746. John Newbery, writer of children's books, publisher (of *Mother Goose* among other titles) and medicine merchant, entered an agreement with Dr James. Newbery had been originally introduced to James by Samuel Johnson. Newbery would manufacture the powders at his premises near to St Paul's Cathedral in London, in return for a half share in the takings. Newbery even included none-too-subtle advertising for the product in his books. In *Goody Two Shoes*, probably written by Newbery in collaboration with Oliver Goldsmith, Goody's father was *'seized with a violent Fever, in a place where Dr James's Powder was not to be had, and where he died miserably'*.

In the 1764 edition of *A Dissertation on Fevers and Inflammatory Distempers*, James claimed that he had sold 1,612,800 doses since patenting the product. According to Newbery's records, he bought 136 gross of packets (19,584 packets) from James in 1769. Even allowing for a publicist's approach to statistics, it certainly seems that sales were high.

Francis Newbery took over his uncle's business and built a new warehouse at 45 St Paul's Churchyard in 1778. He continued to manufacture the powders. The oldest impression in the proof-book preserved in the Stamping Department at Somerset House was the medicine tax stamp appropriated to F Newbery and Sons of Dr James's Fever Powder.

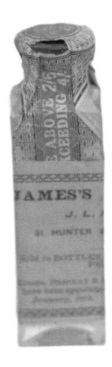

James claimed to have invented his fever powders in 1743, before patenting them three years later. They quickly caused controversy. To acquire a patent, James should have had to prove that he was the sole inventor of the medicine and deposited a precise specification of the mode of production in Chancery. However, his opponents claimed that he had simply adapted William Schwanberg's existing remedy, and that his method for producing this recipe remained unclear. Schwanberg's powder was made by burning shavings of hartshorn or of bones with sulphuret of antimony, and continually raking or stirring them together until the sulphur was burnt off and the powder had become light grey or ash-coloured. Walter Baker, a London chemist, led the charge that James had taken his process of manufacture from William Schwanberg without any payment. James survived this onslaught, winning the argument that his preparation was different from Schwanberg's.

In spite, or perhaps because of, the controversy, James's Powder was extremely popular in the 1700s. Antimonial preparations were generally popular in this period. They were used to treat fevers through diaphoresis (sweating), emesis (vomiting), and purgation and therefore were believed to restore balance in the body. Dr James's Powder was relatively mild in small doses and could produce sweating without vomiting, which was a benefit in comparison to other preparations. However, antimony is a poisonous substance, and can be fatal if taken to excess.

In 1776, Richard Cumberland wrote an ode to James:

O thou, to whom such healing power is giv'n
The delegate, as we believe, of heaven.

Horace Walpole apparently said that he would take the powder if his house was on fire. He also wrote:

> *you may be well in a night, if you will, by taking six grains of James's powder. He cannot cure death, but he can cure most complaints that are not mortal, or chronical.*

O thou, to whom such healing power is giv'n The delegate, as we believe, of heaven

James's Powders were also given to King George III as part of his treatment for an attack of mania in 1788. Recent analysis of a strand of the king's hair revealed high levels of arsenic. Researchers have concluded that this came from contaminated antimony in the Dr James's Fever Powder, prescribed by the king's doctor, to be taken four times daily.

Oliver Goldsmith, author of *The Vicar of Wakefield*, was also a big fan. In 1772, he obtained relief from strangury (a bladder condition) by taking the powder. Although his apothecary had advised against them, Goldsmith also took the powder during his fatal illness in 1774. His apothecary, William Hawes, published an account of Goldsmith's death warning against excessive use of the powders. The issue was still being debated in 1929 when an article in *The Lancet* written by Sir William Hale-White concluded that Goldsmith's death was accelerated by antimony poisoning.

There was other contemporary criticism of the powder. Malcolm Flemyng, a physician, wrote in his *Dissertation on Dr James's Powders* (1760) that physicians should be '*cautious in advising and directing the exhibition of brisk and churlish medicines; lest, while they charitably intend a benefit they do their neighbour irreparable damage*'. Even Samuel Johnson, who wrote '*No man brought more mind to his profession*' also claimed that the ingredients in James's medicines were '*sometimes inefficacious and trifling, and sometimes heterogeneous and destructive of each other*'.

James's patent specification was:

Take antimony, calcine it with a continual protracted heat in a flat unglazed earthen vessel, adding to it from time to time a sufficient quantity of any animal oil and salt well dephlegmated; then boil it in melted nitre for a considerable time, and separate the powder from the nitre by dissolving it in water.

The first independent analysis of the powder was carried out as part of the controversy with Walter Baker. Baker supported his argument with the results of analysis carried out on 30 September 1851 at Mr Erasmus King's Experimental Room at Duke's Court, St Martin's Lane. He had expert witnesses present, and claimed that by carrying out experiments using James's Powder and Schwanberg's he could show that both produced similar results and therefore they were the same powder. James retaliated with evidence from Humphrey Jackson, a chemist, who proved that James's Powder contained mercury, and therefore differed from Schwanberg's.

Pulvis antimonalis or antimony powder was introduced as an official substitute in the 1788 *London Pharmacopoeia*. The formula was one pound of powdered 'Sesquisulphuret of Antimony' and two pounds of shaved horn. This formula was based on analysis by a man called Higgins working in the laboratory at the Society of Apothecaries. However, there was no suggestion through a synonym that this was the same as 'Dr James's Powder'. Chemists and druggists therefore used the term 'Pulvis Jacobi Vera' to signify the real Dr James's Powder from its substitute.

In 1791, a Dr George Pearson carried out his own analysis, publishing the results in the Royal Society's *Philosophical Transactions*. He said that the powder consisted of equal parts of oxide of antimony and phosphate of lime. The formula in the first *British Pharmacopoeia* in 1864, given as

Formula published by Dr George Pearson, 1791

Phosphorated lime, with a little antimonial calx	100.00 parts
Algaroth powder	57.15 parts
Insoluble antimonial calx with a little phosphorated lime	19.85 parts
The same insoluble calx with, probably, a little phosphorated lime	55.00 parts
Waste	8.00 parts
Total	240.00 parts

one part of antimonious oxide and two parts of calcium phosphate, was based on Pearson's analysis.

In 1823, Richard Phillips analysed Dr James's Powder, concentrating on the nature of the oxide in the formula. He concluded that antimony pentoxide was present, and that the presence of this level of peroxide was the significant difference between Dr James's Powder and *Pulvis antimonalis*.

Even in 1869, a Michael Donovan, honorary member of the College of Pharmacy of Philadelphia, was attempting to replicate production of the powder, describing his experiments in full in an article in the *Pharmaceutical Journal*. His conclusion was that James's Powder was prepared by heating bone-shavings over a moderate fire until it was burnt to a black powder. Four ounces of levigated sulphur of antimony was added and stirred until all the sulphurous fumes escaped. The substance was then heated to red hot for two or three minutes, and the contents continued to be raked. They were then described as '*the colour of Bath brick dust*'. After the substance had been powdered and sifted, they were heated at a uniform red heat for an hour. The subsequent white powder was reduced to a fine powder in an earthenware mortar and sifted through a fine silk sieve. Donovan concluded that the process showed that Schawanberg's powders were actually more medically active than James's.

In addition to his fever powder, James patented an 'analeptic' pill which combined the fever powder with pil.rufi (pills compounded of aloes, myrrh and crocus), and gum ammoniacum. The last two ingredients were supposed to be '*dissolved in an underground cave furnished with the conductors of electrical fire*'.

James is also remembered for his three volume *Medical Dictionary*. He was helped in the preparation of it by Dr Johnson, who wrote the dedication, and also much of the main content. Johnson also drew up a four-page pamphlet entitled *Proposals for Printing a Medicinal Dictionary* in 1741. The book's aim was expressed in the proposal:

> *It is not pretended that this Book will make every Reader a complete Physician; but it will be some Recommendation of the Work, if it*

shall enable Mankind to detect the Impostures of confident Pretenders to Physic, and escape those Frauds which are often practised at the Expence [sic] of Life; and shall instruct those who live remote from Physicians.

The first volume was published in 1743, with the second and third following in 1745. The price of the set was £9.6s (£9.30). The total number of pages was close to 4000. Its contents ranged from definitions of different dosage forms, to the use of medicinal ingredients including toads, animal fat and laudanum, to the medicinal use of the word 'abracadabra'.

James's publications also included *Pharmacopoeia Universalis or a New Universal English Dispensatory*, published in 1747, and a *Treatise on Canine Madness*, published in 1760, in which he recommended treating hydrophobia with mercury.

James died on 23 March 1776, aged 71. An advert was placed in the *London Chronicle* on 20 February 1777 to counteract the activities of an unauthorised person who claimed to know the secret of the powders.

Advertising continued to stress the direct link with Dr James himself. In the first half of the 1800s, one of James's grandsons, RGG James, began marketing what he claimed was the original preparation, which had been lost when Newbery changed the formula. A Dr Robert E Robinson of Virginia, USA, also claimed to have the original formula, as it had been given to his father by a Dr Reynolds who was a contemporary of Dr James's son. This formula apparently corresponded with that used by a Mr Adams, who frequently prepared the powder for Dr James. An advert in *The Chemist and Druggist* in May 1860, stated:

We prepare THE POWDER FROM THE ONLY FORMULA OF THE PROCESS EXTANT, which was left in DR. JAMES' own handwriting with our great grandfather, who, as partner and co-patentee with the Doctor, conducted the business of this particular interest.

The same advert also quoted *Dr Graham's Modern Domestic Medicine*: '"*Newbery's James' Powder*" should always be used' (5th edition, page 38). Packets of the powders formed part of the contents of Queen

Victoria's medicine chest in the 1860s.

In 1878, Barclay and Sons, 95 Farringdon Street, London, were appointed as sole wholesale agents for the powders, which were prepared by John L Kiddle, previously of 31 Hunter Street, Brunswick Square.

The powders survived in use just into the 20th century. The last advert placed in *The Chemists' and Druggists' Diary* by Francis Newbery and Sons that mentioned Dr James's Fever Powders and Analeptic pills was in 1906. The final retail price, according to J Sanger and Son's catalogue in 1907, was 2/9d (about 14p).

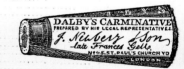

NEWBERY'S NEW GLUTEN CAPSULES. Copaiba, Copaiba and Cubebs, and Copaiba and Citrate of Iron.
Gluten *v.* Gelatine. Gluten as an Envelope Immeasurably Superior.

| Beautifully made; egg-shape. Regular in size. | Contain no air bubbles. More convenient to take. | Smaller than those of other makers, Though containing usual quantity. | Pleasanter in action. Do not cause eructations. |

IF TRIED, WILL BE APPROVED.

OTTLES of 36 Capsules, 2s.; 10s. per doz. Thirteen to the doz. on taking 24 doz. Per 1,000, 14s. All in bottles and subject to the usual Discount.

BRITISH AND FOREIGN MEDICINE WAREHOUSE.

FRANCIS NEWBERY AND SONS,
(ESTABLISHED A.D., 1746.)
45, ST. PAUL'S CHURCHYARD, LONDON, ENGLAND.
Offer to Merchants, Importers, and Foreign Purchasers generally,

Dr. James's Powder.
Dr. James's Analeptic Pills.
Dr. Steers' Opodeldoc.
Steers' Chamomile Drops.
Gell's Dalby's Carminative.
Collins' Cordial Cephalic Snuff.

Direct Shipments of Medicines, &c., are constantly received from America, France, &c., including Jayne's (Dr.) Expectorant, &c., Brandreth's Pills Ayer's Cherry Pectoral, Barry's Tricopherous, Perry Davis' Pain Killer, Radway's Ready Relief, Wright's Pills Winslow's Soothing Syrup, McMunn's Elixir of Opium, Dalley's Pain Extractor, Brown's Bronchial Troches, Allen's Hair Restorer, &c. Dr. Laville's Gout Medicines, Chauten's, Elixir Suisse, Belloc's Charcoal, Blancard's Pills, Grimault's Preparations, Papier Fayard, Papier d'Albespeyres, Eau de Cologne, Lang's Mellissus, &c. &c.
On receipt of TRADE CARD, NEWBERY and SONS *will forward their Catalogue.*

Advertisement reproduced with permission from *The Chemist + Druggist Magazine*, 1868

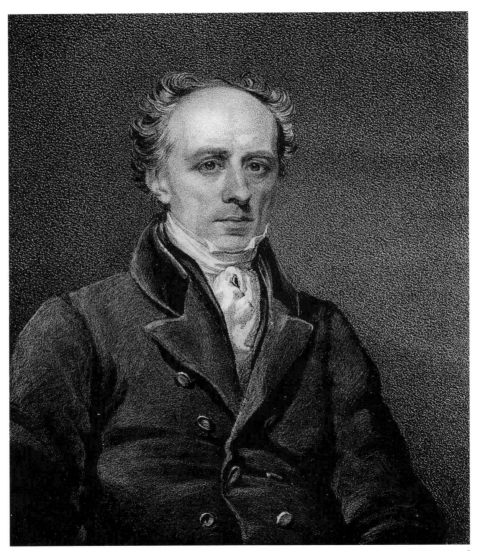

Portrait of Morison from *Morisonia*, 3rd edn 1831 © Royal Pharmaceutical Society

Chapter Thirteen
Morison's Pills

Described by *Punch*, alongside Thomas Holloway, as *'one of the most remarkable pillers* [sic] *of Society'*, James Morison attracted both positive and negative attention from the launch of his pills in 1825 onwards. They have stayed in the limelight among pharmacy historians for many of the same reasons that they originally achieved notoriety: the sheer volume of pills sold, the attendant marketing machine, and the man behind the product.

James Morison was born in Aberdeenshire on 3 March 1770. After some education at Marischal College of the University of Aberdeen, and at Hanau in Germany, he spent around 30 years as a merchant, and travelled widely in Europe, North America, and the West Indies. Having built up significant capital, he returned to Aberdeen to live in a house belonging to George Reid, a partner in a druggist company with a David Souter.

Morison seems to have started work on six different types of pill in 1816, when he lived above these pharmacy premises. It is not clear what prompted him to begin making medicine: was he encouraged by his new insight into the pharmacy business? Did he have inside knowledge of the market as his brother was a doctor? Morison later claimed that the development of his pills was in response to his own long-standing ill health. He related that between the ages of 16 and 50, he saw at least 50 doctors to seek advice on his symptoms, which ranged from total lack of sleep to stiff joints, and from raw flesh to constipation. He tried an impressive range of treatments including vermifuges, cold baths, ether, quinine, mineral waters and surgery. He reported that, at the age of 51, he was so desperately ill that he decided to treat himself. His conclusion was: '*It can then be nothing else but my bad humours, which, from my stomach and bowels, are diffused all over my body. I then rested settled as to that point, resolved to place my confidence in the vegetable medicine as the only rational purifiers of the blood and system*'.

Morison launched six varieties of pill from 1825. Only observers referred to his medicine as Morison's Pills. The man himself called them the Hygeian Vegetable Universal Medicine. There were many similar medicines for sale both before and after Morison. Anderson's Scots Pills were not dissimilar, and had been on the market since at least 1635. However, a major selling point for Morison's pills was his claim that they formed part of an overarching medical theory, the Hygeian system. The system's basis was that all diseases originated from impurities in the blood, and that therefore a medicine that would purify the blood would treat any disease.

Morison's business took off rapidly. He employed a team of agents, known as the Hygeists. They called on clients, advised on treating conditions, supplied the pills, gave lectures on the Hygeian system, and handed out literature. At the start, the fact that these were not medical men was used as a selling point. Hygeists all claimed that Morison's pills had cured them of a particular serious condition. By 1833, the list of salesmen stretched to 24 pages just for England, and there were others in the USA, Ireland, Scotland and Wales.

Morison had started his business in Frith Street, Soho, London, but by 1828, he had built 'The British College of Health' opposite the site of St Pancras Station. This site, 33 Euston Road, housed the college for nearly a century, before ultimately becoming a shelter for the Salvation Army in the early 20th century. It has been suggested that his establishment of the college was an extremely shrewd move. Rather than presenting himself as a manufacturer and salesman, he took on the appearance of a learned society.

Morison attacked the medical establishment and their methods of treating disease, presenting his system of medicine as superior. Morison's criticisms ranged from the reliance on chemicals and mercury, to too close a relationship between medicine and religion. He inevitably gained publicity and many enemies, chief among them Thomas Wakeley, best known as the founder of *The Lancet*.

Morison published *Morisonia*, a collection of his works, in 1829. Stretching to over 600 pages, it was described on the frontispiece as:

> *a complete manual for individuals and families, for every thing that regards preserving them in health, and curing their diseases. The whole tried and proved by the members of the British College of Health, as the only true theory and practice of medicine; and thus furnishing ample testimony that the old medical science is completely wrong.*

" the old medical science is completely wrong "

Morison went on to explain that wounds, bruises, sprains, sores, ulcers, cancers, boils, contracted joints or sinews, aneurisms, sore nipples, scalds, burns, corns, bunions, wens (boils or cysts), hydrophobia, white swellings, poisoned wounds, mortifications, ruptures, stone syphilis, deformities, diseases of the spine, injuries and all mineral and vegetable poisons, could be treated with his medicine, with varying quantities and combinations of, what he had by now narrowed down to, two types of pills.

It seems that Morison retained only two pills (known as number 1 and number 2), as six seemed too unwieldy. The patient was advised to take the two pills in combination in a variety of regimes depending on his condition. For example, bruises and sprains should be treated for a week, at which time they will disappear. The patient should take four or five of pill one, followed by four or five of pill two on the first night, and increase the dose each night by one or two pills. White swellings of the legs would be saved from amputation with one 11/- packet of pills used over a month. The average instruction seems to have been 15–20 pills per day.

The extent of Morison's publicity was immense with images, pamphlets, brochures, almanacs, broadsides, posters and a range of handouts. In 1834, the *London Medical Gazette* claimed:

*We can scarcely go into any street in London in which we do not see
"Morison's Universal Pills for the cure of every disease" staring us
in large letters in the windows of one or more shops.*

Morison based most of this promotional material on testimonials,
predominantly gathered through his network of agents. Morison also
used at least 11 promotional illustrations, with titles including '*Downfall
of the doctors*' and '*Morality of the modern medicine mongers*'. They
were probably handed out as publicity rather than sold.

The sale of the Vegetable Medicine also benefited from promotion as a
treatment for cholera, particular during an epidemic in 1832. Morison
had published a pamphlet in 1825 entitled *A letter addressed to the
honourable the court of directors of the United East India Company
proposing an easy and safe remedy for the prevention and cure of the
Cholera Morbus*.

Morison's recommendations of high dosages marked his pills out from
their competitors. The Hygeian philosophy meant the more pills a
patient took the more impurities would be swept from the blood and
out through the bowels. In fact, Morison's literature warned that if
insufficient pills were taken, the impurities would collect in the bowels
and cause the patient 'uneasiness'. Nevertheless, the high doses were not
without danger. In 1836, John MacKenzie, aged 32, was administered 1000
pills over 20 days by one of Morison's agents. MacKenzie died, and the
agent was severely fined by Morison. In 1837, there were 12 deaths
caused by excessive doses of Morison's pills in York. Cases against
Morison were at a height between 1834 and 1836, and continued until 1839.

Thomas Wakeley used these and many other court cases as evidence
to attack Morison as a visible representative of secret remedies and
quackery. Wakeley also accused the Society of Apothecaries of taking
no action against Morison, even though, by prescribing and compounding
medicines, he was acting as an apothecary.

This negative publicity also appeared in the *London Medical Gazette*, and
non-medical publications such as the *Weekly Dispatch*. In all cases, the
verdict was that the pills had caused or hastened death. However, it was
Morison's agents who were charged. Behind the scenes, Morison paid the

fines, and even awarded the title of 'First Hygeian Martyr' to one of his agents, Joseph Webb, who was convicted in one of the first cases. Morison continued to fight what he saw as a battle to uphold medical liberty.

Morison's notoriety also prompted many poems, songs, articles and images in opposition. John Harkness of Church Street, Preston, had a poem of eight verses, entitled 'The Vegetable Pills', published:

> *Of all the wonders we have read since first the world began*
> *The greatest lately has appear'd and Morrison's* [sic] *the man;*
> *No longer death we need to fear, or labour under ills,*
> *For ev'ry disease is cured by 'The Vegetable Pills'*
> *He says 'they're sure to do it—they're very sure to do it*
> *They're safe and sure to do it are the Vegetable Pills . . .*
> *. . . In short the blind may gain their sight, the dumb may find a tongue,*
> *The lame may quickly run a race, the old again be young,*
> *One dose will make you laugh or cry, the hungry belly fills,*
> *In fact, if you would never die, take the Vegetable Pills.*

At least 25 caricatures were published during the 1830s ridiculing his pills. George Cruikshank featured Morison's pills in a number of his caricatures including *The Fox and the Goose, The Sick Goose and the Council of Health,* and *Morison's Pills—a great reduction on taking a quantity.*

Morison never divulged the exact ingredients for the two pills except that pill number 1 was supposedly a mild aperient, and pill 2 was a purgative. In response to American imitations he stated that only he and his partner '*are privy to the knowledge of the true composition of these medicines;— and that, consequently, any spurious attempt at imitation, from the pretended possession of such a copy, is, and must be, founded on a barefaced falsehood*'.

There have been a number of analyses of the pills over time. An analysis reported in *The Chemist and Druggist* in 1880 showed:

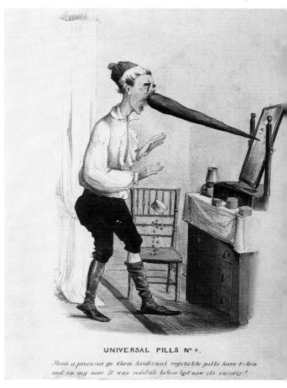

Published by W. Spooner, 1830s
© Royal Pharmaceutical Society

UNIVERSAL PILLS Nº 4.

No. 1 pills: aloes 10g, cream of tartar 5g, senna 5g, made into .13g pills, and rolled in cream of tartar.
No 2 pills: aloes 20g, colocynth 15g, gamboge 15g, jalap 10g, cream of tartar 10g, made into .13g pills and rolled in cream of tartar.

In *Exposures of Quackery* (volume 2), written by the anonymous editor of the *Health Journal* and published in 1896, a slightly different analysis of the pills by Henry Beasley stated:

No. 1—aloes and cream of tartar in equal proportions
No. 2—two parts of gamboge, 3 parts of aloes, one part of colocynth, and four parts of cream of tartar, worked into pills with the aid of syrup.

The writer concluded that there was '*Nothing wonderful or novel about these pills, at any rate, except that one greatly wonders what there is about them to render it necessary for the proprietors of the nostrum to style their emporium the College of Health, or themselves Hygeists*'.

By 1921, MacEwan in *Pharmaceutical Formulas* gave the ingredients for 50 pills (number 1).

Pill number 2 had the same ingredients apart from cream of tartar replacing gamboge, but with greater strengths. These analyses do show that all of the active ingredients are cathartic agents and of vegetable origin.

Formula, 1921	
Aloes	30 grains
Jalap resin	15 grains
Extract of colocynth	15 grains
Gamboge	15 grains
Rhubarb	45 grains
Myrrh	30 grains

It has been suggested that the varying results of the pills' analysis may be attributed to poor quality control in their manufacture; neither size nor ingredients were consistent. This was backed up by evidence at a trial in 1834 when Morison's Pills were accused of causing death. A chemist witness stated: '*the components are occasionally very imperfectly mixed— probably from large quantities being prepared at a time, and the mass not triturated with sufficient care*'.

Morison was 55 years old when he found success. He was particularly keen to expand into France, and moved to Paris in 1834, where he set up a business with a doctor, Dr Lapouge, and a pharmacist, Monsieur

Blain. However, the pills did not sell particularly well. Morison died in a house at Number 2 rue des Pyramides in Paris on 3 May 1840. His sons reported that, at the moment of his death, he was reaching for a box of vegetable pills. He was buried in a family crypt at Kensal Green cemetery.

After Morison's death, his sons Alexander (1809–1879) and John (1812–1886) took over the British College of Health. They continued in their father's footsteps, and also introduced a powder, an ointment, and, in France, a powder to make lemonade. They instigated an award medal, an essay competition, and a publication, *The Hygeist*, first printed in 1842, to print these essays alongside poems and odes. They also presented several petitions to Parliament to promote their pills, including one in 1847 with 20,000 signatures that denounced ingredients in medicines that were not of vegetable origin.

A memorial to Morison, first proposed in 1851, was placed on the College of Health, paid for by penny subscription. *Punch* suggested a slab of stone in the churchyard that contained the most of Morison's late patients, or a memorial made of 'monumental brass' to reflect Morison's character.

The actual memorial consisted of a stone lion mounted on a pedestal, with inscriptions relating to the evils of poisons, the foundations of the Hygeian system, and the petitions presented to Parliament. The monument was erected on 31 March 1856 and remained on the site opposite St Pancras Station until the late 1920s.

By the time of Morison's death in 1840, the pills were on sale in the British Isles, the USA, France and Germany. In 1846, the pills were introduced to Nova Scotia, imported duty free on the request of a member of the Assembly. By the late 1860s, their boom was over and the heavy advertising ceased. They were still sold in the UK until the 1920s and in other countries into the 1930s.

"Shall Morison have a monument? . . . We have no hesitation in saying, by all means let Morison have a monument and we go even further for we beg leave to offer a design which Morisonians are quite at liberty to accept."

Reprinted in *The Chemist and Druggist*, 1952 © Punch

In spite of opposition and legal action, there is no doubt that Morison's pills were phenomenally successful in financial terms. In 1840, Morison left around £500,000 in his will. Thomas Wakeley claimed that Morison paid more than £7000 each year to the Government for the 1$^1/_2$ d medicine duty stamps which had to be attached to his pill boxes. Helfand has calculated that more than a billion pills must have been sold between 1825 and 1849, based on the number of medicine tax stamps used in this period.

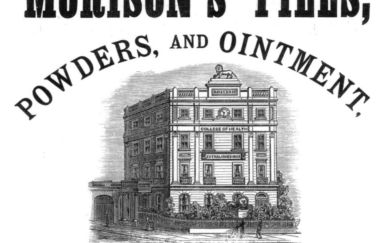

MORISON'S PILLS,
POWDERS, AND OINTMENT,

THE MOST SAFE, EFFICACIOUS, AND PROMPT

VEGETABLE MEDICINE
FOR FAMILY USE.

Compounded of the Purest Vegetable Ingredients only.

SUITABLE FOR ALL CLIMATES AND CONSTITUTIONS.

UPWARDS OF SEVENTY YEARS OF UNINTERRUPTED SUCCESS,

FULL DIRECTIONS FOR USE IN MOST LANGUAGES.

WHOLESALE AT THE
BRITISH COLLEGE OF HEALTH
33 EUSTON ROAD, LONDON.

Reproduced with permission from *Chemists' and Druggists' Diary*, 1901

Chapter Fourteen
Mother Seigel's Syrup

Who was Mother Seigel? According to Audson White (1824–1898), a Yale-educated typewriter manufacturer, Mrs Edith Seigel, a German lady of the Shaker sect, was born at the end of the 1700s and formulated a herbal curative syrup. White acquired the syrup's formula and began to make and sell it in America in 1867. In 1875, Judson entered a deal with the Shaker community of Mount Lebanon, New York State, to buy all of his herbal ingredients from the community which had established its first medical garden in 1820. In the United States, Mother Seigel's Syrup was re-named Shaker Extract of Roots in the late 1800s. However, Judson exported Mother Seigel's Syrup to Britain from 1877 onwards. The syrup was primarily sold as a remedy for dyspepsia (indigestion).

An article in *The Chemist and Druggist* in 1880 explains how the same Mr White attempted to introduce his 'Shaker Extract' to Germany and Turkey by distributing pamphlets and placing advertisements in newspapers. *The Pharmaceutische Zeitung* published an account of a pharmacist in Dresden who was approached by White to act as an agent for his product. The pharmacist went straight to his local paper and persuaded them to publish a paragraph warning the public against the medicine. The Police of Public Health seized 500 bottles and 60,000 pamphlets as Mr White's German representative did not hold the necessary trading licence. In Turkey, members of the

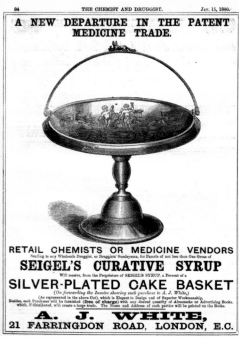

Reproduced with permission from *Chemists' and Druggists' Diary*, 1880

Formula, 1891

Tincture of capsicum	10 drops
Tincture of gentian	30 drops
Fluid extract of taraxacum (dandelion)	2 drachms
Fluid extract of euonymus	1 drachm
Fluid extract of cascara	3 drachms
Oil of sassafras	5 drops
Oil of wintergreen	2 drops
Rectified spirit	2 drachms
Borax	20 grains
Concentrated compound decoction of aloes	2 ounces
Treacle	to 4 ounces

Dissolve the oils in the spirit and the borax in the first five ingredients. Add the spirit to the decoction, then the borax solution. Mix.

Pharmaceutical Society of Constantinople '*deplored the popularity of this unwholesome product*' and resolved to alert editors of newspapers that carrying adverts for it risked public safety.

What was all the fuss about? In *The Universal Memorandum Book and Diary for 1879–1880*, published by White, price one halfpenny, are many testimonials for the syrup. The successful treatments reported include cases of rheumatism, bronchitis, piles, liver complaints, inflammation of the kidneys, skin diseases, and improvements to people suffering from asthma and consumption. The product's contents were given as five alkaloids with soporific, laxative, sudorific, diuretic and alterative properties.

According to White, the remedy contained *Iris versicolor* (blue flag iris), *Stillingia officinalis* (queen's root), *Taraxacum officinale* (dandelion), *Juglans regia* (royal walnut), *Gaultheria procumbens* (checker berry), *Hydrastis canadensis* (yellow root), *Euonymus atropurpureus* (spindle tree), *Actaea racemosa* (black cohosh), *Gentiana rubra* (gentian) aloe, *Capsicum annuum* (pepper), and *Lignum sassafras* (sassafras wood). Borax, simple syrup, hydrochloric acid and powdered Spanish pepper were then added. An early 20th century advertisement claimed that the remedy was '*compounded of roots, barks and leaves*'.

However, a less complimentary description was given by a Dr Theodor Petersen of Frankfurt, amazingly as part of an advert for the syrup in a German newspaper. He described the medicine as '*a dark-brown, emulsion-like, turbid, watery extract, of fresh smell, bitter taste and acid reaction*'.

The formula was published in *The Chemist and Druggist* on 21 November 1891.

The formulation seems to have changed a number of times over the 20th century with different plant extracts in varying quantities. However, a pharmacist working in the 1920s remembered the contempt that his apprentice master had for proprietary medicines, with Mother Seigel's Syrup as a particular example. A customer who asked for the preparation was told '*to buy a horse physic ball and a tin of cattle treacle; go home and stir with a kettleful of hot water to end up with half a gallon or more of Mother Seigel's syrup*!'

The medicine and its formula last appears in *Martindale* in its 26th edition (1972) as Mother Seigels [*sic*] Syrup.

In 1909, a 3-fluid ounce bottle of Mother Seigel's Curative Syrup cost 2/6d (about 13p). The bottle's wrapper was printed '*A cure for impurities of the blood*' and '*A cure for dyspepsia and liver complaints*'. The circular with the bottle raged against dyspepsia:

The symptoms mentioned above are the smoke of the fire of indigestion—a fire that will eat out your very vitals and sap your strength and vitality. For it can't be too often repeated that indigestion is the root of a great deal of evil; the origin of a great many disorders which no man quite understands how he came by. And why this is can easily be explained. Disease is poison; its symptoms are the manifestation of the poison. Indigestion creates many dangerous poisons, and is therefore the cause of many diseases.

So let us get rid of the smoke by putting out the fire, and purify our blood and system with Mother Seigel's Syrup, which will sweep away the poisons and make us healthy and strong.

Formula, 1909

Dilute hydrochloric acid (B.P.)	10 parts by measure
Tincture of capsicum	1.7 parts by measure
Aloes	2 parts
Treacle	60 parts
Water	to 100 parts by measure

Formula, 1972

Boiling water extractive of capsicum	0.24%
Boiling water extractive of *Chimaphila umbellata*	2.92%
Boiling water extractive of *Cimicifuga* (black cohosh)	4.4%
Boiling water extractive of colocynth	0.56%
Boiling water extractive of *Taraxacum* (dandelion)	1.84%
Boiling water extractive of gentian	0.56%
Boiling water extractive of orris	2.8%
Boiling water extractive of *Stillingia*	4.56%
Boiling water extractive of walnut leaves	9.12%
Boiling water extractive of *Phytolacca* (poke root)	2.72%
Boiling water extractive of *Leptandra* (black root)	3.64%
Aloes	1.24%
Hydrochloric acid	1.64%
Light kaolin	0.72%

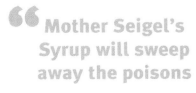

" Mother Seigel's Syrup will sweep away the poisons "

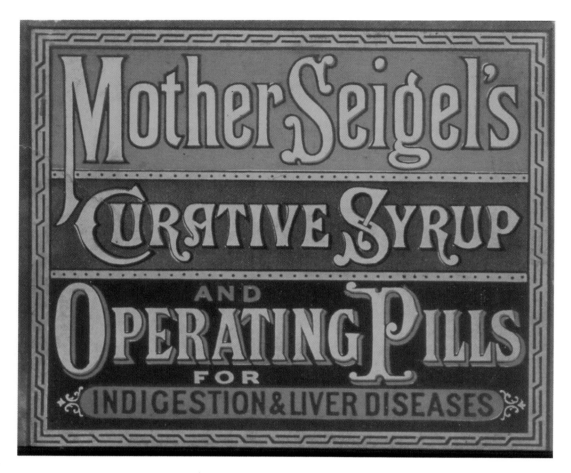

More precisely, the claim through the product's advertising was that the '*highly concentrated, purely vegetable compound*' had '*a specific action on the stomach, liver, and kidneys*'.

A Judson White established a company, AJ White Ltd, in London in 1884. He also transferred his New York headquarters to the UK, and the original New York side of the business became a subsidiary. The British business was incorporated as a limited liability company at 17 (later 39) Farringdon Road, London. The company remained American-owned. White held 56% of the shares, and most of the directors were American. By the end of the 1800s, production branches of AJ White had been established in Madrid, Lille, Barcelona, Sydney and Cape Town. An advert from the early 20th century stated:

The unrivalled success of Mother Seigel's Syrup as a stomach and liver remedy, and digestive tonic, accounts for its world-wide popularity. For forty years it has been the unfailing family friend in thousands upon thousands of homes, and to-day it is the most popular household remedy in sixteen different countries!

Adverts for Malt Cough Balsam, Plasters, Ointment, Operating Pills and Syrup were produced in German, Dutch, English and French.

However, a subsequent business White established collapsed and left him in significant debt. He therefore sold AJ White Ltd in 1897 for £960,000. White died in 1898.

A new company also called AJ White Ltd was registered in London with £1 million capital. Amazingly, £929,000 of this was goodwill. According to Tony Corley's research, the net profit of the company, after large expenditure on advertising, was said to be £90,000 each year.

The advertising expenditure in Britain was £150,000 per year, but profits fell after 1897, perhaps because White was no longer involved in the company. An advert in *The Chemists' and Druggists' Diary* in 1900 claimed that the syrup was the '*most popular and effective dyspepsia cure and nerve tonic known, used in 572,000 British households*'. However, when the remedy was first sold in Britain in 1877, the company's annual profits were £89,000. By 1903/4, they had fallen to £32,000, and a year later they were only £13,000. A representative of the American

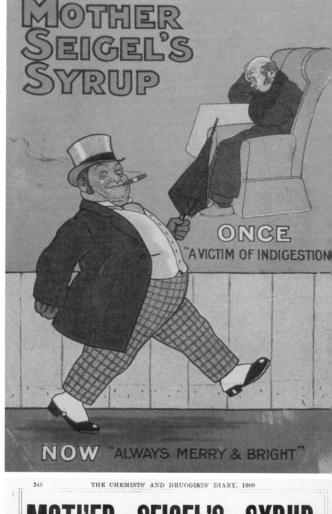

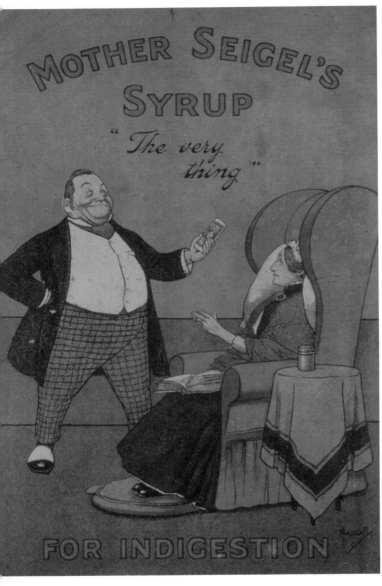

© Museum of Brands

shareholders visited London to see what action should be taken. They claimed there were irregularities, and the capital was written down to £300,000.

By 1907, the shareholders and company directors were British. In the same year a subsidiary was established which would not show any connection with the White name – Menley and James Ltd. It went on to manufacture pharmaceutical specialities including Aspirin, Laxol, Calomex and Gonorex. The company rented the ground floor of 39 Farringdon Road until 1916 when it bought a factory at Coldharbour Lane, Camberwell, Southwark, London.

In 1920, AJ White Ltd relocated from Farringdon Road to 64 Hatton Garden, which from 1927 was called Menley House. In 1940, it moved to join Menley and James Ltd at Coldharbour Lane.

In 1927, AJ White Ltd was appointed by Smith Kline & French Co. Inc., USA, to distribute its products under licence. This continued until 1956, when the then Smith Kline & French Laboratories Inc. acquired AJ White Ltd and Menley & James Ltd as UK subsidiaries. AJ White Ltd was renamed Smith Kline & French Laboratories Ltd and relocated to Welwyn Garden City, Hertfordshire.

However, the story of Mother Seigel's Syrup became uncoupled from AJ White Ltd in 1957. For three years from this point, the syrup was supplied by CF Abel Ltd, and then from 1961 until 1967 'Mother Seigel's Digestive Syrup' was marketed by Fassett and Johnson, Oxford Works, Worsley Bridge Road, London SE26. In 1968, it appears in the *Buyers Guide of The Chemist and Druggist Yearbook* supplied by Marns, Thomas and Co., and then it disappears. All a long way from the kitchen of a German lady in the 1700s.

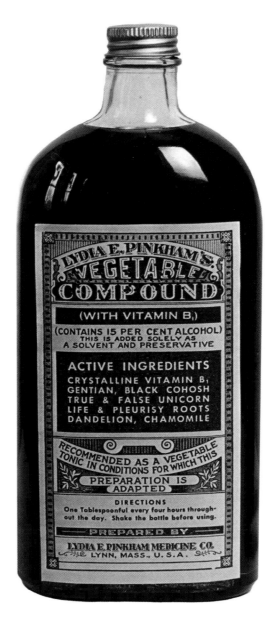

Chapter Fifteen

Lydia E Pinkham's Vegetable Compound

We'll drink a drink a drink
To Lily the Pink the Pink the Pink,
The saviour of the human race.
For she invented medicinal compound,
Most efficacious in every case.

T his is the opening chorus of a song made famous in the 1960s by a group of singers called Scaffold. But was there such a person? There was, indeed, and her name was Mrs Lydia Estes Pinkham. The 'medicinal' compound was, in fact, a vegetable compound. She was one of the first women entrepreneurs making a fortune from her products by using the power of advertising to target women, offering a cure for their afflictions.

Lydia was born on 9 February 1819 in Lynn, Massachusetts, the 10th child of William and Rebecca Estes. Her father had been a shoemaker, the owner of a saltworks, a gentleman farmer and had made a fortune from real estate. At the age of 16, Lydia joined the Lynn Female Anti-Slavery Society. She graduated from Lynn Academy, became a schoolteacher and, in 1843 was

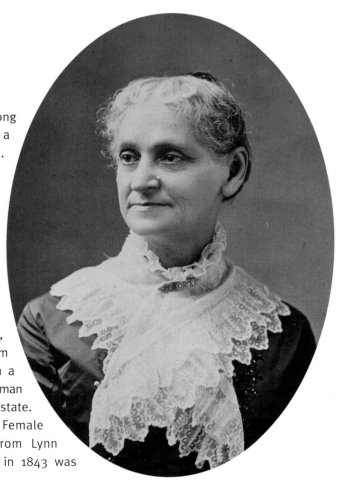

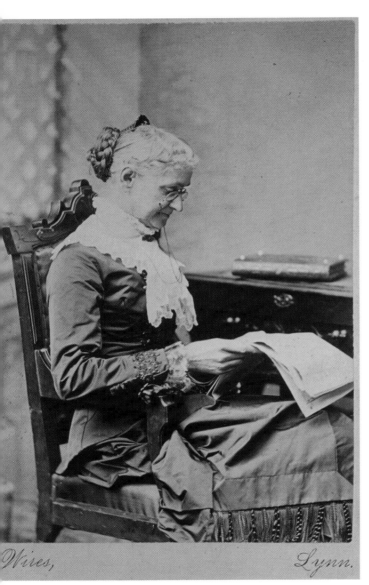

Wires, *Lynn.*

elected secretary of the Freeman's Institute where she met, and soon after married Isaac Pinkham, a 29-year-old widower and shoe manufacturer. They had four children, Charles, Daniel, William and Aroline. Isaac was not a good businessman and tried many trades but was caught up in the failure in 1873 of Jay Cooke, a New York banking house, and lost most of his finance. He never recovered from the effects and died in 1889. By 1875 the family were struggling and it was at this time that Daniel thought of selling his mother's cure for women's ailments.

Some years before, Isaac had received a formula for a medicinal compound as part payment for a debt. Lydia had always been interested in herbal cures, especially those from John King's *The American Dispensatory*. It is not clear where her formula came from, perhaps a combination of the two sources, but she made up bottles and gave them to friends for 'female complaints'. This was the compound that would be sold through the family business, set up in 1876, named The Lydia E. Pinkham Medicine Company. Lydia would become famous throughout America.

Lydia died in 1883. Charles's wife, Jennie Pinkham, became the nominal head of the company. Daniel and William had both died in 1881. Aroline had married Will Gove in 1882 and equally divided her half-share in the company with him. When Charles died in 1900, the Goves seized control and Will Gove became president and general manager. Jennie's son Arthur insisted that all letters addressed to Mrs Pinkham should be delivered to his mother, not to the factory, and then set up a rival company selling exactly the same formula as the Vegetable Compound but called it Delmac Liver Regulator. On the label was a picture of Charles Pinkham *'known throughout the country by druggists as the manufacturer of "Pinkham's Vegetable Compound"'*. The result was that it was agreed not to market the new product and Arthur became a member of the board of Pinkham's.

Will Gove died in 1920. After some dispute, a new board of directors was formed of three Pinkhams and three Goves. Family disputes continued and in 1937 an injunction was granted which forbade the Goves to interfere with the business. In 1968 the business was sold to Cooper Laboratories which moved manufacturing to Puerto Rico. At the time of writing, Numark Laboratories of Edison, New Jersey, market a product named Lydia Pinkham's Herbal Liquid Supplement and Time of Your Life Nutraceuticals of St Petersburg, Florida, produces a product named Lydia's Secret.

Lydia E Pinkham's Vegetable Compound was a product containing vegetable extracts in alcohol that made it as strong as a fortified wine. It was advertised as *'A sure cure for Prolapsus Uterus or Falling of the Womb'*, and for *'all weaknesses of the generative organs of either sex'*.

> **all weaknesses of the generative organs of either sex**

A reproduction of one of her advertisements in *Pharmacy in History* states:

> *Lydia E. Pinkham's Compound is a positive cure for all those Complaints and Weaknesses so common to our best female population.*

> *It will cure entirely the worst forms of Female Complaints, all Ovarian troubles, Inflammation, Ulceration, Falling and Displacements of the Womb, and the consequent Spinal Weakness, and is particularly adapted to the Change of Life.*

> *It will dissolve and expel Tumours from the Uterus in an early stage of development. The tendency to cancerous tumours there is checked very speedily by its use. It removes faintness, flatulency, destroys all cravings for stimulants, and relieves weakness of the stomach. It cures Bloating, Headaches, Nervous Prostration, General Debility, Sleeplessness, Depression and Indigestion.*

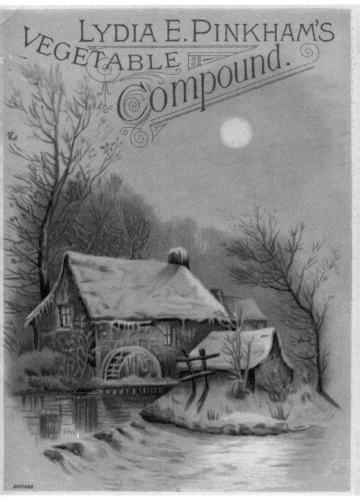

LYDIA E. PINKHAM'S
VEGETABLE COMPOUND

IS A POSITIVE CURE

For all those painful Complaints and Weaknesses so common our best female population.

It will cure entirely the worst form of Female Complaints Ovarian troubles, Inflammation, Ulceration, Falling and Displments of the Womb and the consequent Spinal Weakness, an particularly adapted to the Change of Life.

It will dissolve and expel Tumors from the uterus in an e stage of development. The tendency to cancerous humors the checked very speedily by its use. It removes faintness, flatule destroys all craving for stimulants, and relieves weakness of stomach. It cures Bloating, Headache, Nervous Prostra General Debility, Sleeplessness, Depression and Indigestion.

That feeling of bearing down, causing pain, weight and back. is always permanently cured by its use.

It will at all times and under all circumstances act in harm with the laws that govern the female system. For the cur Kidney Complaints of either sex, this Compound is unsurpasse

Lydia E. Pinkham's Vegetable Compound is prepare Lynn, Mass. Price, $1.00. Six bottles for $5.00. Sent by ma the form of Pills, also in the form of Lozenges, on receipt of p $1.00 per box, for either. Send for pamphlet. All letter inquiry promptly answered. Address as above.

No family should be without LYDIA E. PINKHAM'S LI PILLS. They cure Constipation, Biliousness, and torpidity of Liver. 25 cents per box.

LYDIA E. PINKHAM'S
BLOOD PURIFIER

This preparation will eradicate every vestige of Humors the Blood, and at the same time will give tone and strength t system.

It is far superior to any other known remedy, for the cure o diseases arising from impurities of the blood, such as Scro Rheumatism, Cancerous Humor, Erysipelas, Canker, Salt Rh and Skin Diseases.

SOLD BY ALL DRUGGISTS.

Compliments of

Cressler & Greenawalt,
Druggists,
Chambersburg, Pa.

© Royal Pharmaceutical Society
(both pages)

That feeling of bearing down, causing pain, weight and backache, is always permanently cured by its use.

It will at all times and under all circumstances act in harmony with the laws that govern the female system. For the cure of Kidney Complaints of either sex this Compound is unsurpassed.

Lydia produced a four-page guide featuring her cures. This was initially distributed on a door-to-door basis but then her son, William, paid $60 to have the pamphlet printed in full on the front page of the *Boston Herald*. Within two days wholesalers were contacting them for supplies.

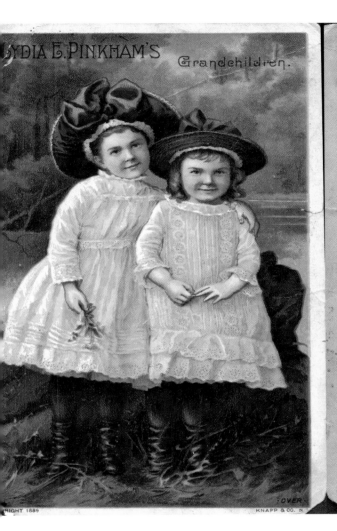

Encouraged by this they spent thousands of dollars on advertising, which by the end of the 19th century rose to $1 million a year.

Another strategy was, in 1879, to put a 'benevolent' lady's face on the packaging and it was decided to use Lydia herself. By 1881 annual sales had reached $200,000 and Lydia's face was known throughout the USA. By 1941 it was estimated that $40 million had been spent on printing likenesses of Lydia's face.

From 1879 advertisements invited women to write about their complaints, confidentiality guaranteed. No men ever saw these letters because all of the office staff were women; men were only employed for heavy jobs in the warehouse. Lydia would reply personally to the letters. However when she died in 1883, the practice was continued by Jennie Pinkham and advertisements continued to insinuate that Lydia was still alive. In 1905 *The Ladies Home Journal* reprinted a Pinkham advertisement that advised women to write to Mrs Pinkham for advice, and alongside it a photograph of Lydia's tombstone showing that she had died 22 years earlier. Sales slumped.

In 1900 eight men were arrested while distributing Pinkham leaflets, which were said to be 'obscene literature' because of references to prolapsed uterus, menstrual disorders and leucorrhoea. Wordings were changed to less outrageous claims but pamphlets were still used to extol the virtues of Pinkham products over other medicines.

Trade improved in the 1940s but fell in the 1950s. Advertising was discontinued with the takeover by Cooper Laboratories in 1968.

In *Female Complaints; Lydia Pinkham and the Business of Women's Medicine* there is a reference to a formula, said to be in Lydia Pinkham's own hand, that was found in the Radcliffe College Library at Harvard University.

More Secret Remedies commented that a bottle they examined was in a package marked 'Made in U.S.A.' and contained nearly 7 fluid ounces. It contained 19.3% alcohol and '*constituents usual in vegetable preparations . . . and no evidence was obtained of any active principle except a trace of a bitter substance . . .*'. Arthur J Cramp of the American Medical Association's Department of Propaganda was against quack medicines and, as a result of this analysis, suggested that it should be classed as a 'medicated liquor' as it did not contain sufficient medicament to prevent it being used as a beverage. The company reformulated the compound by increasing the proportion of the original ingredients and adding dandelion, chamomile, liquorice root and gentian.

At the time of writing, Numark Laboratories Inc., Edison, New Jersey, market Lydia Pinkham's Herbal Liquid Supplement, which contains: motherwort,

Formula, possibly mid-1800s

Unicorn root (*Aletris farinose*)	8 ounces
Life root (*Senecio aureus*)	6 ounces
Black cohosh (*Cimicifuga racemosa*)	6 ounces
Pleurisy root (*Asclepias tuberosa*)	6 ounces
Foenugreek seed (*Foenum graceum*)	12 ounces
Alcohol (18%), sufficient quantity to produce	100 US pints

gentian (*Gentiana lutea*), Jamaican dogwood (*Piscidia erthrina*), pleurisy root (*Asclepias tuberosa*), liquorice (*Glycyrrhiza glabra*), black cohosh (*Cimicifuga racemosa*) and dandelion (*Taraxacum officinale*).

Also available is a product by Time of Your Life Nutraceuticals, St Petersburg, Florida, named Lydia's Secret for Lydiapinkham.org. Said to be 'based on' the original formula, it has these listed ingredients: black cohosh root, dandelion root, pleurisy root, chastetree berry, false unicorn root, Jamaica dogwood bark, gentian root, vitamin E, vitamin B6, magnesium, zinc.

This chapter has concentrated on the liquid version of Lydia E Pinkham's Vegetable Compound but it was also available in the form of pills or as lozenges. The company also produced Lydia E Pinkham's Blood Purifier Pills, '*far superior to any other known remedy for the cure of all diseases arising from impurities of the blood, such as Scrofula, Rheumatism, Cancerous Humours, Erysipelas, Canker, Salt Rheum and Skin Diseases*'.

Lydia and her family were members of a temperance society. There may have been some justification for her use of the original ingredients taken from John King's *The American Dispensatory* but this did not stop her from producing what must have been a pleasantly warming, highly alcoholic drink that made the consumer feel that the compound was, indeed, working.

We started with a song; we will end with an un-attributed American rhyme:

Oh! It sells for a dollar a bottle,
And it cures all manner of ills;
And it's more to be recommended
Than Carter's Liver Pills.

The Author acknowledges the heavy reliance on the article by WA 'Bill' Jackson: 'Who Was Lily the Pink?', published in the *Pharmaceutical Historian* in July 1998, volume 28, number 2, pages 22–28.

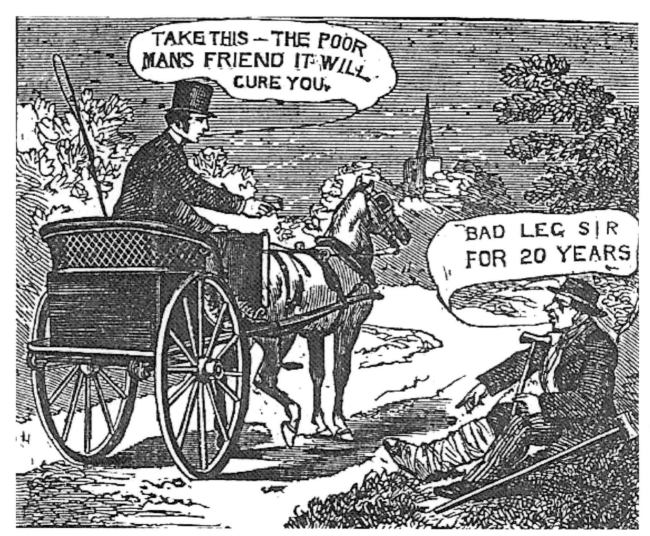

Chapter Sixteen
*P*oor Man's Friend Ointment

D r Roberts's Poor Man's Friend Ointment was first developed by Dr Giles Lawrence Roberts in Bridport, Dorset, in the 1790s. He had been born at West Bay, Bridport, on 21 April 1766, where his father was reputedly a pilot and innkeeper. The story goes that Roberts tried a number of trades before studying medicine. He returned to Bridport where he established a pharmacy in 1788, aged 23. In 1794, he went to London to study anatomy and midwifery at Guy's and St Thomas' Hospital. He returned to Bridport for a second time in 1795, and expanded his work to that of a surgeon, apothecary and accoucheur or male-midwife. In April 1797 he was given the degree of Doctor of Medicine from King's College, Aberdeen.

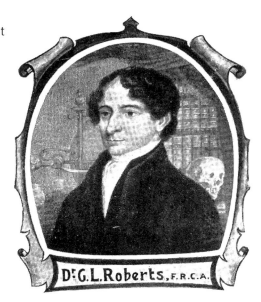

Dr.G.L.Roberts, F.R.C.A.

© Royal Pharmaceutical Society

Poor Man's Friend Ointment was reputed to have been the second best-selling patent medicine in Britain in the early 1800s. In 1824, the ointment was apparently sold by 140 chemists across England including six in London and one in Dublin. Dr Roberts also developed Pilulae Antiscrophulae or pills to treat scrofula, which were supposed to be taken with the ointment when eruptions were present.

A major promotional tool for the ointment was a series of booklets, *The Annual Mentor or Cottages Companion presented gratuitously by G.L.*

G. L. Roberts, M.D.
1788—1834.

———

Beach & Barnicott
1834—1860.

———

James Beach
1860—1903.

———

Beach & Co.
1903—

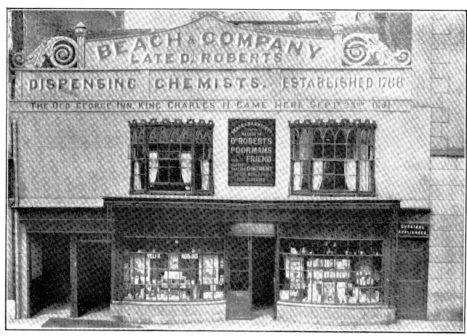

© **Royal Pharmaceutical Society** *Roberts M.D. Proprietor of that Celebrated Ointment called the Poor Man's Friend*, which appeared from 1829 until at least 1883. The booklet usually had a cartoon on its cover. The remainder of the publication included testimonials and warnings against substitute products alongside notes on the ointment and the pills.

Dr Roberts had a variety of other interests. He established his own private museum collection of curiosities. He was a lay preacher. In 1824, he published *Sentimental and Humorous Essays by G.L.Roberts M.D. Proprietor of that Celebrated Ointment called the Poor Man's Friend*. In 1832, Roberts was the first person in Bridport to install gas lighting.

Dr Roberts died on 16 September 1834, aged 69. He left his business, including all the stock in hand, buildings and the recipes for his medicines to his two apprentices and close friends, Thomas Beach and John Barnicott, who carried on the business in partnership. Beach and Barnicott continued to trade together from Roberts's original premises. They are listed in *Pigot and Co's Directory of Dorsetshire*, 1842, on East Street, Bridport. The pharmacy was housed in a building dating from

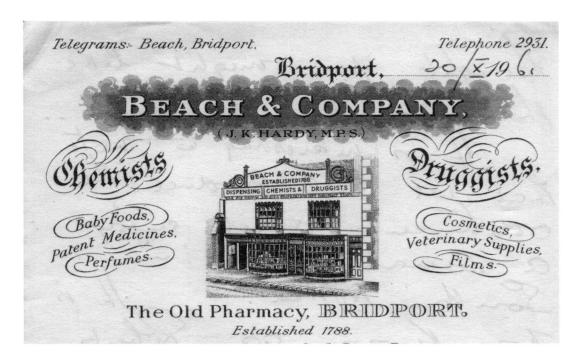

Telegrams:- Beach, Bridport.

Telephone 2931.

Bridport, 20/X 196.

BEACH & COMPANY,

(J. K. HARDY, M.P.S.)

Chemists

Druggists.

Baby Foods,
Patent Medicines,
Perfumes.

Cosmetics,
Veterinary Supplies,
Films.

BEACH & COMPANY
ESTABLISHED 1788
DISPENSING CHEMISTS & DRUGGISTS

The Old Pharmacy, BRIDPORT.

Established 1788.

the 1500s. As a public house called the George Inn, King Charles II was supposed to have sought refuge there on 23 September 1651 to hide from Cromwellian soldiers.

Thomas Beach was born in 1800 at Portchester, son of William and Elizabeth Beach. He married Mary Ann Berry Barnicott at Bridport on 21 June 1826. They had at least nine children. By 1834, John Barnicott had married Catherine Oliver. They had at least three children.

When Thomas Beach retired in 1860, his son James Beach continued the business. John Barnicott subsequently died on 18 October 1865, with a personal estate valued around £14,000. James Beach was recorded in the 1881 census at 1 Market Place, Bridport. He was mayor of Bridport in 1885 and stayed in the town until his death on 14 October 1924, aged 93. In 1903, James's son, Thomas Edgar Beach, had taken over the family business. He continued to trade both as Beach and Barnicott Ltd and as Beach and Co. TE Beach had qualified as a pharmacist in 1888. The business remained in the Beach family until 1947 when it was sold to a Mr Hardy. Beach died on 20 February 1955, aged 93. The premises continued as a pharmacy into the 1970s.

> **" the ointment of many virtues "**

One advert for Poor Man's Friend Ointment referred to it as '*the ointment of many virtues*'. Each box of pills had the image of Hercules killing the Hydra. Testimonials that featured in adverts for both Poor Man's Friend Ointment and Roberts' Alterative Pills showed that they were being used to treat scurvy, scurf, '*scorbutic in the face*', '*scorbutic eruption in the leg*', sore and inflamed eyes, and running leg wounds. Adverts claimed that the ointment should be used to treat cuts, scalds, chilblains, scorbutic eruptions, burns, bruises, ulcers, pimples in the face, weak and inflamed eyes, piles, fistula, gangrene, and '*is a specific for those Eruptions that sometimes follow Vaccination*'. Advertising continued to tie Roberts's two products together: '*Much of the success of this ointment depends on using the alterative pills at the same time*'. An advert from 1901 recommended the ointment for wounds and skin diseases and promoted the alterative pills to purify the blood and as '*a gentle aperient and perfect liver pill*'.

The medicine was sold for '*headaches, bruises, gout etc*' into the 20th century. It was still on sale in South Africa in the 1960s.

The ointment's formula first appeared in the 22nd edition of *Martindale* in 1943. The Pharmacy and Medicines Act of 1941 had made it compulsory to disclose the formula of all preparations sold for medicinal use. The entry for Poor Man's Friend quoted the packaging as saying '*For ulcerated sore legs (even if of twenty years' standing), and wounds and skin eruptions, burns, scalds, chilblains, etc.*'.

DR. ROBERTS' CELEBRATED MEDICINES

THAT EXCELLENT OINTMENT CALLED THE
POOR MAN'S FRIEND,

Is confidently recommended to the Public as an unfailing remedy for Wounds of every description, and a certain Cure for ULCERATED SORE LEGS, even if of twenty years' standing.

CUTS   BURNS,
Scalds,   Bruises,
CHILBLAINS   ULCERS
Scorbutic   Eruptions
Pimples in   the Face,
Weak and   Inflamed Eyes.
Piles & Fistula,   Gangrene.

And is a Specific for those Eruptions that sometimes follow Vaccination.
In Pots at 13½d.; 2s. 9d.; 11s.; and 22s. each.

DR. ROBERTS'S,
PILULÆ ANTISCROPHULÆ,
OR ALTERATIVE PILLS.

Proved by more than SIXTY YEARS' successful experience as an invaluable Remedy for that distressing complaint called SCROPHULA, Glandular Swellings, particularly those of the Neck, &c. They open the obstructed pores, expel all superfluous humours on the Skin, and are one of the best alteratives ever compounded for purifying the Blood and assisting Nature in all her operations. They are efficacious also in Rheumatism, and form a mild and superior FAMILY APERIENT, that may be taken at all times without confinement or change of diet.

Sold in Boxes at 13½d.; 2s. 9d.; 4s. 6d.; 11s. and Family Boxes 22s. each.

By the late Dr. ROBERTS's Will, Messrs. BEACH and BARNICOTT, (who have been confidentially intrusted with the preparation of his Medicines for many years past) are left Joint Proprietors of the Poor Man's Friend, Pilulæ Antiscrophulæ, Larwill's Pills, Medicated Gingerbread Nuts, &c., &c., with the exclusive right, power, and authority to prepare and vend the same.

The increasing demand for these Medicines has excited the cupidity of some unprincipled persons, who shamefully tamper with the health and comfort of others for the advantage of a trifling gain to themselves. The Proprietors anxiously caution the public against the effects of such COUNTERFEIT PREPARATIONS, to put off which many artful means have been resorted to. No Medicines sold under the above names can possibly be genuine unless '*Beach and Barnicott, late Dr. Roberts, Bridport,*' is engraved and printed on the Stamp affixed to each package. Each pot of the Ointment has '*Poor Man's Friend, prepared by Beach & Barnicott successors to Dr. Roberts, Bridport.*'

However, the ointment's original formula remained a mystery until 2003 when its recipe, having been discovered in the Roberts's original shop in an envelope marked 'private', was sold at auction. Bridport Museum bought the recipe which showed that the ointment was made from lard, fine English beeswax, calomel (mercurous chloride), sugar of lead, salts of mercury, zinc oxide, bismuth oxide, Venetian red, oils of rose, bergamot and lavender.

Formula, 1943

Mercury subchloride	3.5%
Lead acetate	1.255%
Red powder	35%
Perfume	0.175%
Bees wax	7%
Lard	7.5%

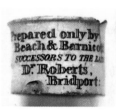 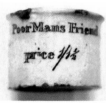 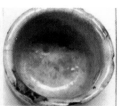 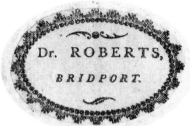

© Bridport Museum

The ointment was sold in distinctive earthenware pots, each about 4cm high and 4.5cm in diameter. The pot would be covered with a parchment cover as its lid. The earliest ones had blue transferred text with '*Poor Man's Friend, price 1/1½*' on the front and '*Prepared only by Dr Roberts, Bridport*' on the reverse. Later jars said '*Prepared only by Beach & Barnicott successors to the late Dr Roberts, Bridport*'. There are some surviving larger pots, simply transfer-printed '*Poor Man's Friend*' which were first produced in the late 1850s or early 1860s. By the early 20th century, the only change to the lettering was that it was printed in black. The ointment continued to be sold in the same pot until the 1920s. It was later marketed as Roberts' Ointment and sold in glass jars.

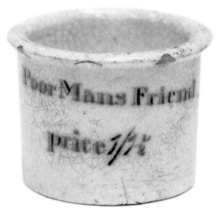

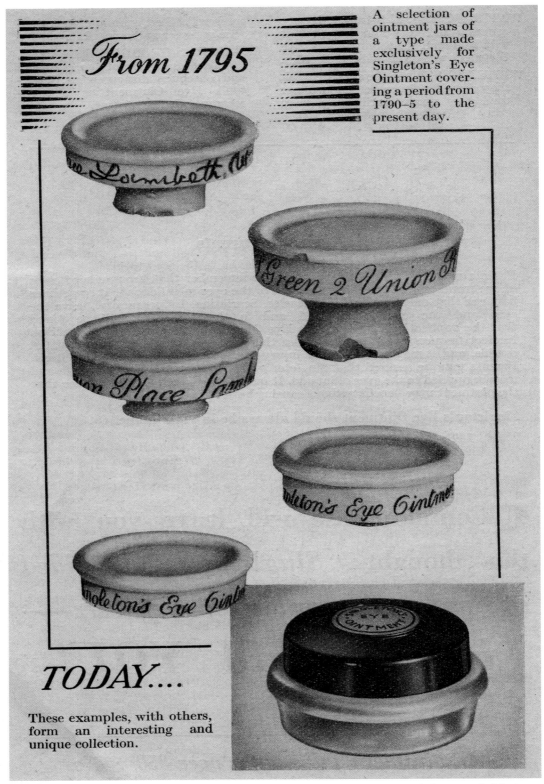

From 1795

A selection of ointment jars of a type made exclusively for Singleton's Eye Ointment covering a period from 1790-5 to the present day.

TODAY....

These examples, with others, form an interesting and unique collection.

Chapter Seventeen
Singleton's Eye Ointment

Singleton's Eye Ointment was one of the most enduring proprietary medicines. According to the company's own booklet the ointment was first made in the reign of Elizabeth I in about 1596. The original formula was prepared by a Doctor Thomas Johnson who was also a botanist and who gave his name to the botanical genus *Johnsonia*. He also translated the works of Ambrose Paré, physician to the French monarchy. In 1644, he died from the effects of a wound received while fighting for the Royalists during the Civil War.

In his will Dr Johnson left his ointment recipe to a gentleman named George Hind who, in turn, passed the recipe to his son William Hind. William gave the recipe to his daughter as a wedding present when she married Thomas Singleton. The Singletons moved into a house in Lambeth Butts, at the time a suburb of London. The picture shows a photograph of a print of Lambeth Road as it appeared in 1670 and the position of the house where it stands today is marked with a cross. Now just called Lambeth, the address of the house is 210 Lambeth Road, and is situated very near to the Headquarters of

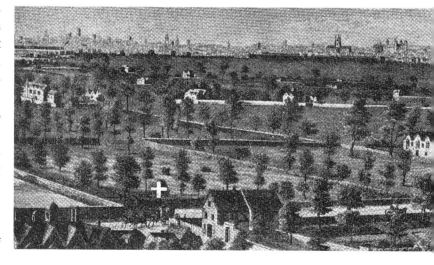

the Royal Pharmaceutical Society. Singleton's Eye Ointment was manufactured here until 1972.

Thomas Singleton died in 1779 and left the recipe to his son William, and it was under William's proprietorship that the ointment became widely known. In 1799 he received a testimonial from the War Office, signed by the Duke of York, bearing testimony to the great value of Singleton's Eye Ointment which had been ordered for use in the British Army while in Egypt 1798 – 1800, during the campaign against Napoleon Bonaparte. Large numbers of British soldiers whose eyes had been injured by the hot desert sand in Egypt were '*perfectly cured by its use*'. William Singleton gave the recipe to his daughter Selina on her marriage to Timothy Folgham. In 1816, she died and bequeathed the recipe to be shared equally by her five children. The eldest child William Singleton Folgham administered the business until his death in 1826 when the administration passed to the second child, Selina.

In 1825, Selina Folgham had married Stephen Green. Her fifth share passed to him in a marriage settlement. He purchased the rights of two of the children and, as the other two had been confined to a lunatic asylum, he agreed to pay an annuity for each until their death and obtained their rights. He took full possession of the company in 1848.

SINGLETON'S
GOLDEN EYE OINTMENT

KNOWN TO THE PUBLIC UPWARDS OF 200 YEARS AS A CERTAIN CURE FOR

INFLAMED EYES, WEAK SIGHT, SORE EYES, SCORBUTIC ERUPTIONS, PILES, BRUISES, &c.

SINGLETON'S GOLDEN EYE OINTMENT has the testimony and patronage of many of the most skilful Oculists and Physicians, who are constantly in the habit of using it.

Dr. BABINGTON recommended the use of SINGLETON'S GOLDEN EYE OINTMENT in the most virulent cases of inflammation, and said "NOTHING ELSE WOULD BE OF USE."

The eminent Oculists, Dr. WARE and Dr. ALEXANDER, were well known to use SINGLETON'S GOLDEN EYE OINTMENT.

CAUTION !—None offered for sale can be genuine unless "SINGLETON'S GOLDEN EYE OINTMENT" is engraved on the Government Stamp and round the Pot, and the Bill of Directions signed, STEPHEN GREEN, 210 Lambeth Road, London, S.E.

Advertisement reproduced with permission from *Chemists' and Druggists' Diary*, 1882

The proprietorship remained with the Green family until 1967 when it was taken over by Fordham Laboratories Ltd at the same Lambeth address. By 1972 it had passed into the hands of Northern Pharmaceuticals Ltd, in Bradford and was finally discontinued in 1974.

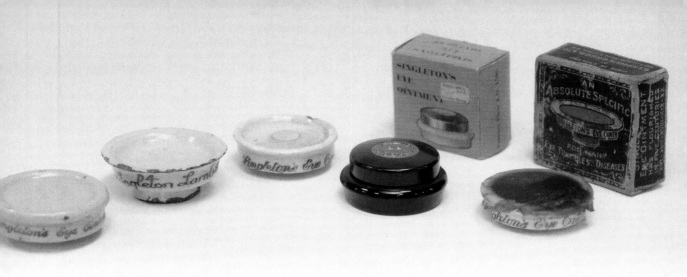

The famous glazed ceramic pedestal pot made its appearance in about 1700 as an item of delftware. Many people have believed that these containers were some form of stopper, but, as the illustration shows, the cavity was filled with ointment and covered with parchment, which was tied on with twine. Each pot held about 55 grains (approximately 3.5 grams). Application of the ointment was with the finger, or later with the aid of a glass rod.

The pots bore the name of the current owner. Also illustrated is an early pot from Singleton with the address as Lambeth Butts (1700s), a later Singleton pot, a Folgham pot and a Green pot.

Until 1892 the ointment, in its pedestal pot, came simply wrapped in a leaflet. In 1892 the ointment was boxed and an article from *The Chemist and Druggist* in July 1892 states that:

> the proprietor of Singleton's Eye Ointment, Mr Stephen Green, of 210 Lambeth Road, is putting up his very well tried remedy in a somewhat new form. The quaint old pots are still used, but they are not now wrapped up in the old handbill with which they have been heretofore enveloped, and they are now supplied in half dozen boxes, for counter sale, as shown in the engraving.

In 1909 Singleton's Eye Ointment was written about in *Secret Remedies*:

> The price charged was 2/- (10p) for a pot containing about 55 grains (approx. 3.5 G).

On the outer package the ointment was described as '*an absolute specific for all Eye Troubles and Diseases*'. An enclosed leaflet stated:

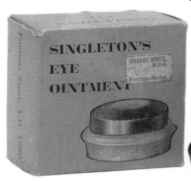

It cures Weak Sight, Inflamed Eyes, and all disorders of the Eyelids from whatever cause arising . . . Singleton's Eye Ointment requires great skill in making, and is composed of costly ingredients. One pot will cure you . . . The Ointment also cures Piles and Scorbutic Eruptions.

By the 1950s it was packed in a plastic pot, finally being packed in a tube.

In the 1950s the company produced a leaflet. It gave advice on the prevention and treatment of eye troubles, how to '*take care of your eyes and never strain them*' and advocated '*prevention was better than cure*'. The leaflet then gives a dictionary of eye troubles. It does not actually state so, but gives the impression that Singleton's ointment will treat all of these conditions. But it is careful to choose its words and treat conditions that may be associated, for example, redness of the eyelids '*which may be associated with Astigmatism or Blurred Vision*'.

The formula of the ointment changed little over most of its life. However, some early entries of the formulation in medical publications proved to be totally incorrect.

The earliest suggestion for a formula for the ointment was given by Dr JA Paris. He surmised that it contained Sulphuret of Arsenic, also known as orpiment, that is arsenic sulphide, in a base of lard or spermaceti ointment. Henry Beasley accepted this surmise and recorded in his *Druggist's Receipt Book* of 1866, that the recipe was Orpiment (Yellow Arsenic Sulphide) mixed with lard to the consistency of an ointment.

The formulas from both these eminent gentlemen were found to be incorrect. A more correct formula appeared in *Cooley's Practical Receipts* of 1864. He writes:

According to Dr Paris, this compound consists of lard medicated with orpiment (native yellow sulphuret of arsenic). There appears, however, to be some mistake in this, as that sold us under the name had nearly the same composition as the Ointment of Nitric Oxide of Mercury of the Pharmacopoeia. It did not contain even a trace of either arsenic or sulphur. The action of this nostrum, and the reputation which it has required, fully justified this conclusion.

The ointment was scientifically analysed for the 1909 edition of *Secret Remedies*. Analysis gave the formula as red mercuric oxide 7.4% in a base that contained a mixture of beeswax, lard, Japan wax and coconut oil.

It finally states '*The assertion that such an ointment "requires great skill in making" is absurd and as to the costliness—one-ninth of a penny*' (0.05p).

Pharmaceutical Formulas was a publication by *The Chemist and Druggist* and gave formulas for preparations that pharmacists could prepare, including proprietary preparations. *Pharmaceutical Formulas*, 1929, quoted Singleton's Golden Ointment as '*Red Precipitate Ointment (that is Red Mercuric Oxide Ointment), 30 grains to the ounce (6%), prepared with a peculiar fat, say goose fat. It is exceedingly well made, the powder being very finely divided*'.

Martindale, 1943, quoted the ointment as: '*for many eye troubles and diseases – the standard remedy which has outlived the centuries. Contains Red Mercuric Oxide 5.45% w/v*'.

> the standard remedy which has outlived the centuries

In *Martindale* 1967 the manufacturer was Fordham Laboratories Ltd, still at 210 Lambeth Road and the formula was red mercuric oxide 5%.

By *Martindale* 1972 the product with the same formula had moved to Northern Pharmaceuticals Ltd, Bradford, and Singleton's Eye Ointment finally disappeared as a product name in 1974.

The name Golden Ointment or Golden Eye Ointment was adopted by many companies who created their own brands. Indeed, the

Pharmaceutical Journal Formulary of 1904 included 44 eye ointments containing either yellow mercuric oxide or red mercuric oxide, three of which bore the synonym of Golden Ointment and nine Golden Eye Ointment. Yellow mercuric oxide was prepared by an interaction between mercuric chloride and sodium hydroxide, and red mercuric oxide by heating mercurous nitrate until acid vapours ceased to be evolved. The oxides are identical in formula but the yellow was thought to be more suitable for eye ointments as the particle size was smaller.

The description Golden Eye Ointment lives on. The latest product, at the time of writing, to bear the name, produced by Typharm, does not contain red mercuric oxide and it is not gold-coloured. It now contains dibromopropamidine isethionate BP 0.15% w/w, and costs £4.95 per tube.

Mercuric oxide ointment was a very suitable preparation for eye troubles; indeed, it is still used for that purpose, at the time of writing, in Australia, France and the USA. The 'pedestal pot' has become a very desirable artefact to antique collectors.

Chapter Eighteen
Steedman's Soothing Powders

*J*ohn Steedman was born at Barnes, Surrey, in July 1786, the son of Thomas Steedman. Thomas was a member of the Carpenters' Company, becoming its Master in 1776. John and two of his business associates, Robert Faulconer and Frederick Arthur Crisp, also became Masters of this guild. John started work as a chemist and druggist at 5 Keens Row, Walworth, London, in 1812. He began to make soothing powders for teething babies early on in his career. There is one story that the formula was approved by a friend who was a physician. Sales were good, and by 1839 he arranged for the medicine duty stamps to be engraved with his name (known as 'appropriated' stamps). By 1843, he opened a bank account with the Bank of England.

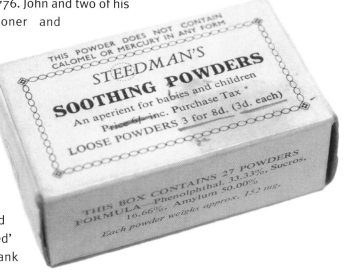

Steedman was one of the Pharmaceutical Society's founder members in 1841. His certificate was number 153. In 1843, Steedman took Robert Stephen Faulconer as his business partner. Faulconer was also an early member of the Pharmaceutical Society, a chemist and druggist, and had married one of Steedman's six daughters. The retail business was known as Steedman and Faulconer until its closure in 1875, and one of Steedman's enduring products was Faulconer's worm powders.

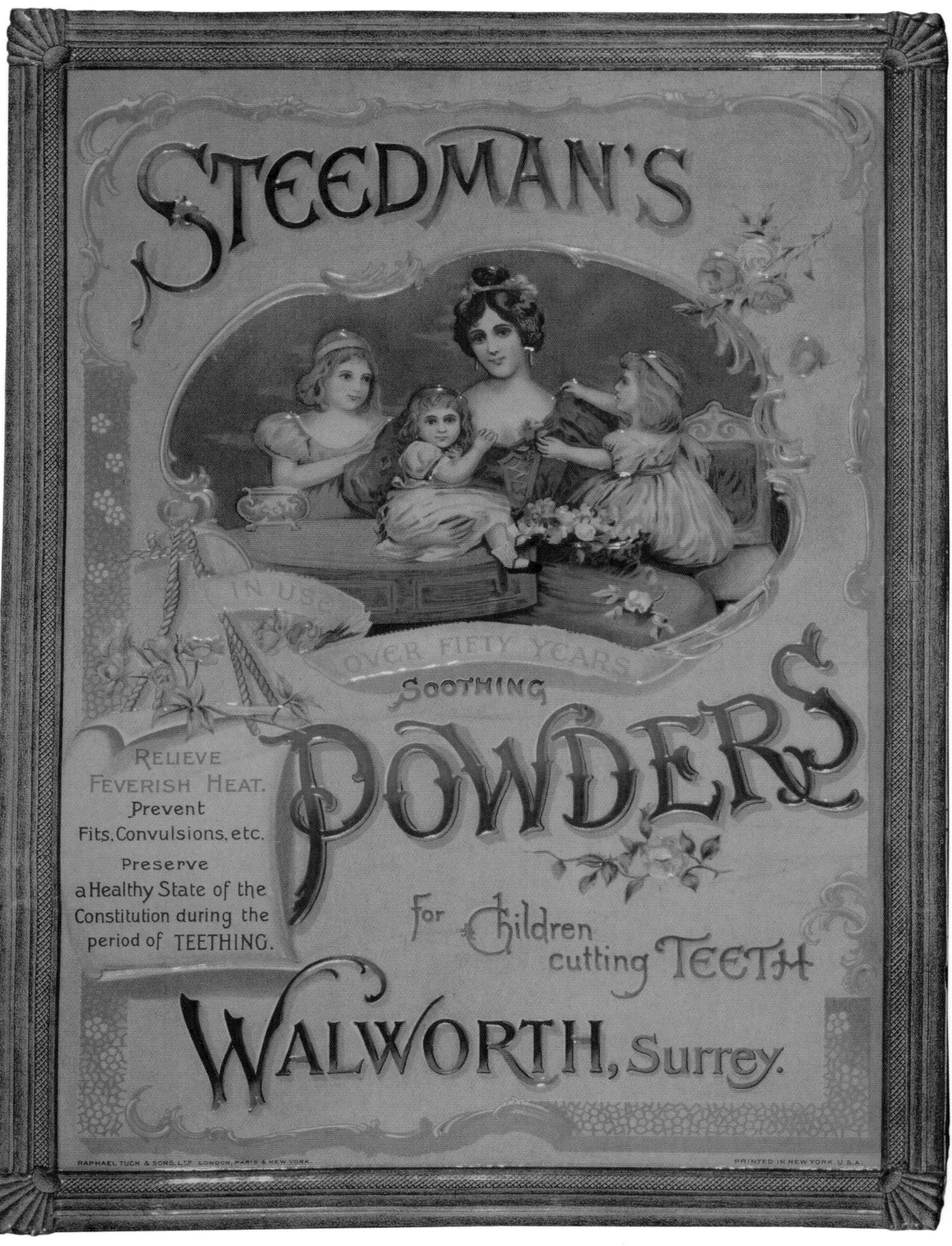

STEEDMAN'S

IN USE

OVER FIFTY YEARS

Soothing

POWDERS

RELIEVE
FEVERISH HEAT.
Prevent
Fits, Convulsions, etc.
Preserve
a Healthy State of the
Constitution during the
period of TEETHING.

For Children
cutting TEETH

WALWORTH, Surrey.

RAPHAEL TUCK & SONS, LTD, LONDON, PARIS & NEW YORK.   PRINTED IN NEW YORK, U.S.A.

However, the partnership agreement between the two specifically reserved the proprietorship of Steedman's Soothing Powders to John Steedman.

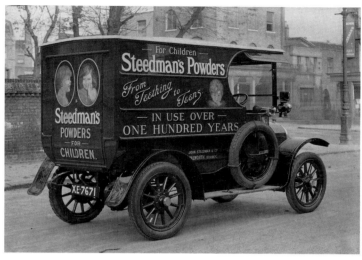

Steedman died on 17 November 1846 and left his property equally between his six daughters. There is a street named after him in Southwark. His wife, Leah, continued the business with Faulconer until the original partnership agreement expired in 1857. At this point her half-share in the business passed to Faulconer. Mrs Steedman died in 1876. The retail pharmacy had closed in 1875, and the fixtures, plate-glass shop front and goodwill of the business were given to Mr WF Smith, pharmacist, of 280 Walworth Road. Faulconer died in 1878.

© **above and opposite:**
Royal Pharmaceutical Society

One of Steedman's daughters, Sarah, married a Fellow of the Royal College of Physicians. Their son, Frederick Arthur Crisp, trained as a pharmacist, and passed the Pharmaceutical Society's Major examination in April 1873. He was manager of the Steedman and Faulconer pharmacy from 1873 to 1875, and then was general manager of John Steedman and Co. Crisp, who was both mayor and a justice of the peace in Godalming, died in 1922.

The circular enclosed in each packet of Steedman's Soothing Powders at the beginning of the 20th century stated:

The good effects of these Powders during the period of Teething have now had Fifty Years' Experience, during which time Thousands of children have been relieved annually from all those distressing symptoms which children suffer while cutting their teeth—viz. Feverish Heats, Fits, Convulsions, Sickness of Stomach and Debility, accompanied with Relaxation of the Bowels, and pale and green motions, or Inflammations of the Gums.

. . . the striking superiority both in the health and strength of those

> **make this MUCH-VALUED MEDICINE more generally known**

children who have taken the soothing Powders during the period of Teething has induced the Proprietor to make this MUCH-VALUED MEDICINE more generally known by this advertisement.

Crisp's daughter, Marion, married Arthur Rust Hunt. Their sons George Rust Hunt and Edmund Crisp Hunt both qualified as pharmacists, and took over management of the Steedman business in the 1920s. At this date, the company, although primarily known for Steedman's Soothing Powders, was also still selling Steedman's Rhubarb and Ginger Pills, Steedman's Whooping Cough Powders, and Faulconer's Worm Powders. In 1939, an article in the *Pharmaceutical Journal* described the business as having '*a large staff of happy girl workers*'. The existing deed of the business still stated that only a lineal descendant of John Steedman could be a partner in the firm.

Steedman's factory and business premises at 270 and 272 Walworth Road stood on the actual and adjoining site of John Steedman's original pharmacy and house. The premises were erected in 1858. Number 270 was the retail chemist's shop and home of Robert Faulconer. Number 272 was built as a house for Steedman's widow. It also contained the premises for making and distributing the powders.

Formula, 1909	
Calomel (mercurous subchloride)	27%
Sugar	22%
Maize starch	50.5%
Ash	0.5%

John Steedman and Company was taken over by Scott and Bowne in 1969. Scott and Bowne, although established in 1888 as an independent company, were taken over by Beecham Group Ltd in the mid-20th century, but retained its name. The 28th edition of *Martindale*, published in 1982, was the last to include a Steedman's product – Steedman's Teething Jelly. Scott and Bowne was dissolved in 1996.

The first insight into the preparation's formula is its analysis published in *Secret Remedies* in 1909. The average weight of one powder was 2.8 grains (0.18 g). The advised dose was one third of a powder for infants between one and three months, half a powder for three to six months and one powder for children above that age, but no more than one powder. The estimated cost of the ingredients in a 2/9d packet was one eighth of a penny.

However, the company disputed the ingredients revealed by *Secret Remedies*, saying that the analysis was both incomplete and inaccurate. At an inquiry into proprietary medicines before a select committee in 1913, John Arthur South, manager of Steedman and Co., stated that the Soothing Powders had had only one change in their formula between their original production and 1913, and this was predominantly to remove opium from the medicine. However, when questioned as to whether giving a child the advertised *'one powder a day'* would actually be harmful to a child, the company's analytical chemist, Dr Wilson Hake, said *'Well, no mother would be likely to give a powder for a long period'*. In answer to the question *'But there is no instruction or caution that the dose is not to be repeated too frequently?'*, Hake had to admit that there was not. John South admitted that Steedman's had refused to sell the powders in Argentina, Uruguay, and Australia because these countries' regulations stated that the presence of calomel in the medicine had to be declared, and this would alarm the public who might think that this was a dangerous ingredient.

The powders still contained mercury until the 1940s. The last appearance of mercury in the formula published in *Martindale* is in 1943 (22nd edition). By 1955, the mercury had been replaced with phenolphthalein, a purgative.

Steedman's Soothing Powder last appeared in *Martindale* in its 27th edition in 1978, alongside Steedman's Nappy Cream and Steedman's Teething Jelly. All three products were sold by Scott and Bowne. Each powder of 152 mg contained phenolphthalein 33.33%, sucrose 16.66% and starch 50%.

Although the formula of the powders was a closely guarded secret in the 1800s, this did not stop an intense battle between Steedman's and their rival Stedman's over the safety of their respective remedies. Stedman's Teething Powders were established by the 1860s. The company was

Formula, 1943	
Mercurous subchloride (calomel)	26.7%
Powdered ipecacuanha	2.2%
Sugar	17.8%
Starch	53.3%

Formula, 1955	
Phenolphthalein	32.61%
Powdered ipecacuanha	2.17%
Sugar	21.74%
Starch	43.48%

STEDMAN'S
TEETHING POWDERS

1/1½ and 2/9 per Packet. TRADE MARK GUM LANCET 1/1½ and 2/9 per Packet.

THE Proprietor of the above now supplies vendors with a pamphlet styled "The Nursery Doctor," of which *The Chemist and Druggist*, June 1880, says —"As the author has had a special experience in this branch of practice, his hints may be expected to be trustworthy;" and of which the *Monthly Magazine of Pharmacy* also says—"Chemists selling Stedman's Powders would do well to secure a supply of the book for their counters." Where agents do not care themselves to prescribe, the proprietor is confident his pamphlet will increase their business, and where doctors are distant and difficult to get at, reliable Nursery Medicines are justly esteemed.

The pamphlet will be indented and sent for enclosure upon instructions. Mind the brand.

STEDMAN'S TEETHING POWDERS.

THE ANALYTICAL INSTITUTION.

54 HOLBORN VIADUCT, E.C.
LONDON, 29th Nov., 1877.

REPORT ON THE TEETHING POWDER PREPARED BY MR. JAS. STEDMAN, HOXTON.

I hereby certify that I have purchased a sample of STEDMAN'S Teething Powder, and have, at the request of the Proprietor, subjected it to Analysis for Morphia or Opium in any form.

I am enabled to state that I found the sample in question to be absolutely free from Morphia, or any other Alkaloid or constituent of Opium.

Thus STEDMAN'S Teething Powder is favourably distinguished from similar preparations.

ARTHUR H. HASSALL, M.D.

Advertisement reproduced with permission from *The Chemist + Druggist Magazine*, 1884

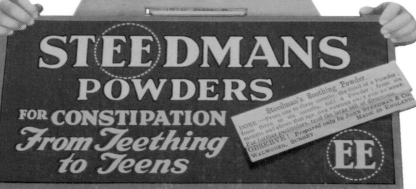

based in East Road, Hoxton in East London. An advert in *The Chemist and Druggist* in 1868 made it clear that the product had gained an extensive sale '*on its own merits*', the suggestion being that the company was attempting to counter any claim that they were profiting from Steedman's popularity. The company appealed to pharmacists that their powders were much cheaper than comparable preparations. By 1868, Stedman's had agents across London, and also in Northampton, Boston (Lincolnshire), Chorley (Lancashire) and Dover (Kent). Stedman's selling point to the public was that their teething powders contained no morphia or opium. An article in *The Chemist and Druggist* in 1886, included a letter from Arthur H Hassall MD of the 'Analytical Institution', 55 Holborn Viaduct, London, with the results of his analysis of Stedman's Teething Powders. The advert stressed that the medicine was not a scheduled poison, and therefore '*vendors need be under no apprehension of the pain, trouble, and censure connected with most inquests, the occasional result of fatal doses of Patent Medicines*'. However, the analysis published in *Secret Remedies* showed the powders to contain calomel or mercurous subchloride, which was obviously a substance that would cause concern among customers.

Steedman's adverts in the second half of the 1800s go to great pains to distinguish themselves from Stedman's.

Observe!! Always with two EE's in the word STEEDMAN, and that the Medicine is prepared ONLY AT WALWORTH, SURREY; also that each SINGLE POWDER has the name and address above.

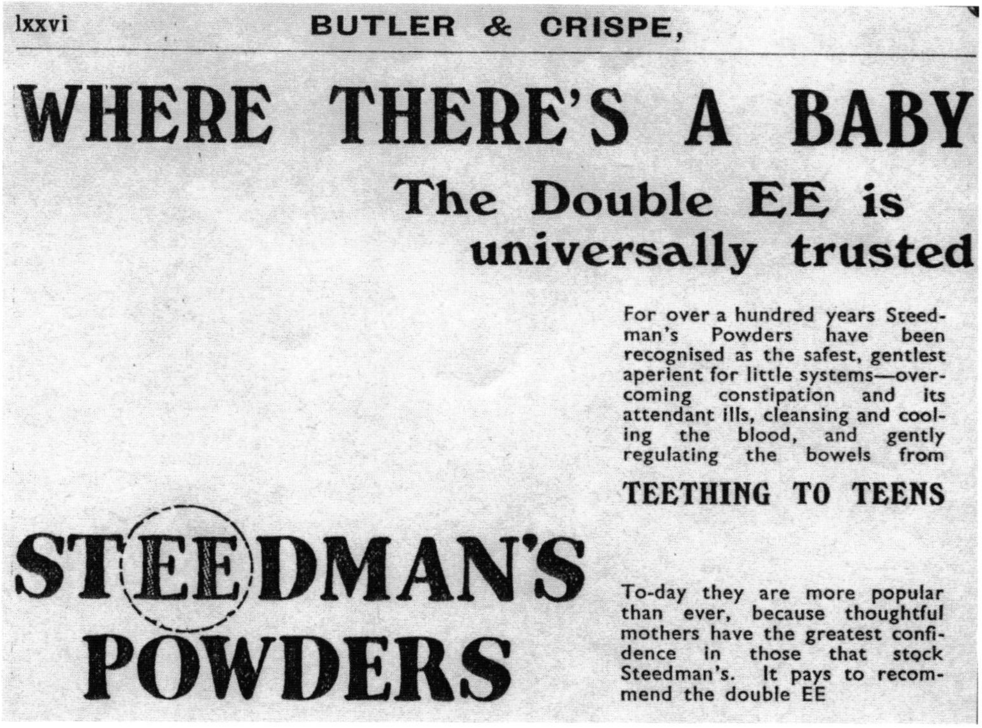

lxxvi
BUTLER & CRISPE,
WHERE THERE'S A BABY
The Double EE is
universally trusted
For over a hundred years Steedman's Powders have been recognised as the safest, gentlest aperient for little systems—overcoming constipation and its attendant ills, cleansing and cooling the blood, and gently regulating the bowels from
TEETHING TO TEENS
STEEDMAN'S
POWDERS
To-day they are more popular than ever, because thoughtful mothers have the greatest confidence in those that stock Steedman's. It pays to recommend the double EE

© Royal Pharmaceutical Society

The rest of the advert has the double 'e' underlined throughout. This same advert (date unknown) says that the powders can be taken with a little moist sugar for the youngest children, placed on the back of the infant's tongue. It is also stated that the medicine will be effective for children long after they have been teething, even up to nine or ten years old.

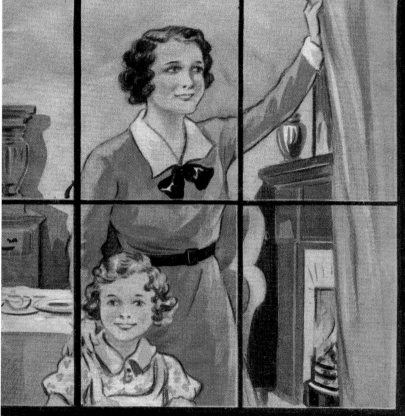

In Every Home

Health Notes
Tasty Dishes
Life Stories

A HELPFUL REFERENCE BOOK
For Everyday Use in Every Home

Chapter Nineteen
Dr William's Pink Pills for Pale People

Although Dr William's Pink Pills for Pale People were originally patented in 1886 by Dr William Frederick Jackson, a physician who practised in Brockville, Ontario, their future success in the market place on both sides of the Atlantic was almost entirely due to the efforts of another Canadian – George Taylor Fulford, uncle of Charles Edward Fulford, inventor of Bile Beans.

Fulford was born in Brockville on 8 August 1852. After a period of study at a local business college and intermittent jobs as a railway and steamship ticket agent and a wholesale jobber of coal, oil and imported goods he finally became an apprentice in his brother William's drug store. In due course he passed through the Ontario College of Pharmacy and in 1879, when his brother decided to move to Chicago, Fulford took over the store and became a successful businessman manufacturing and selling patent medicines. In June 1890 he purchased Jackson's patent for the paltry sum of $53.01 plus the government purchase fee and immediately set about establishing a market for the product both nationally and internationally.

© *The Chemist + Druggist Magazine*, 1893

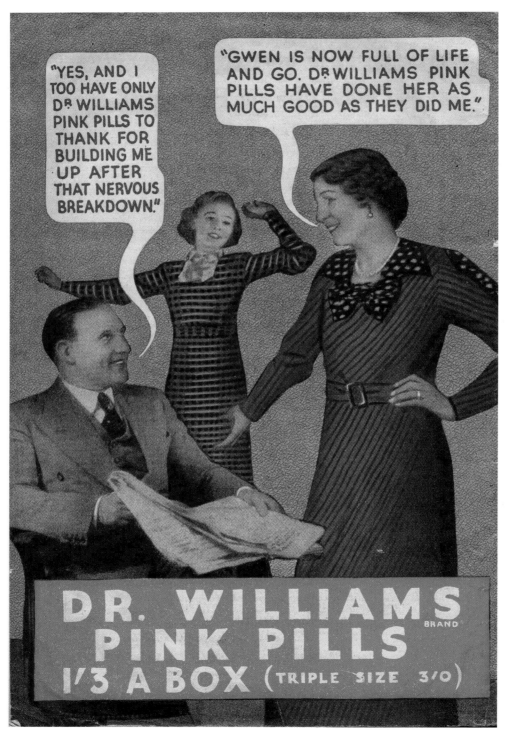

Aided by the fortuitous coincidence of an influenza epidemic in 1891/1892 and original and effective advertising costing in the region of $300,000 a year, sales of the product in 1892 had mounted to a million boxes a year in Canada alone. Fulford then formed a partnership with Willis Tracy Hanson based in Schenectady, New York, to market the pills in the USA. In January 1893 he employed John Morgan Richards based in London as agents for the UK. Within months and aided by advertising contracts with nearly 200 weekly newspapers and a team of 60 men distributing five million pamphlets countrywide, sales in the UK had exceeded all expectations. The operation quickly expanded with the establishment of offices and agencies in France, Holland, Belgium, Italy, Greece, South Africa, Australia and China. In most cases the pills were made in Canada and exported in bulk for packing in the various markets.

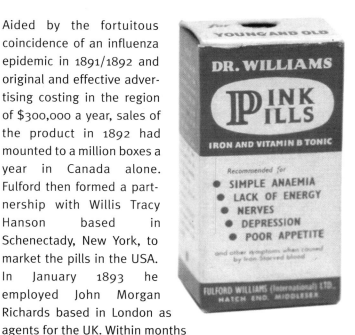
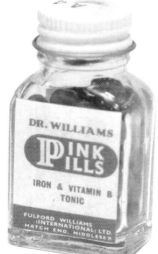

Despite his growing international reputation, Fulford chose to remain in Brockville where he became an active and prominent member of the community. He served on the town council for 12 years and for 10 of these he was Chairman of the Finance Committee. He sat on the boards of a number of corporations and was a benefactor to a number of charities. He donated a pulpit and altar to the Methodist Church as well as generous contributions to the YMCA, the Brockville Rowing Club and General Hospital. At a personal level he liked to pay for the education of a bright child who had been brought to his attention. In 1900 he was appointed to the Canadian Senate where he used his expertise in international business on various committees investigating competition and import duties. Fulford died following injuries sustained in a motor accident on 15 October 1905. In just 15 years he had risen from being a small time owner of a drug store to a wealthy, internationally known business magnate with a seat in the Canadian Senate.

Fulford had a relatively simple approach to success. In an interview with *The Chemist and Druggist* in 1893 he stated, '*Three things are essential. First, you must have a good thing; secondly, you must advertise it cleverly; and, third, you must have lots of money to back it up with*'. He certainly practised what he preached; in the UK alone in 1893 he was spending £3000 per month on advertising and this rose to a staggering £200,000 per annum by 1900.

Fulford was very conscious of his reputation and that his product should not be regarded as a quack remedy. In his very early pamphlets he claimed that the pills were '*a thoroughly scientific preparation, the result of years of careful study on the part of an eminent graduate of McGill Medical College, Montreal, and Edinburgh University, Scotland ... They supply in a condensed form, the substances actually needed to enrich the blood and restore the nerves*'. This was regarded as '*Utter Bosh!*' by the anonymous editor of the *Exposures to Quackery* in 1895. Nevertheless the product became so acceptable in society circles in London that in 1901 *The Chemist and Druggist* reported:

> quite a Society boom just now in Pink Pills for Pale People . . . People in good society who ten years ago, or even one year ago, who would not have dreamed of using any advertised medicine have recently become quite fond of the pills which Mr Fulford brought over from Canada seven years ago. The reason for this, it is said, is that the fact has leaked out that a certain foreign Royal Family has to be ranked amongst the pale people whose countenances have been improved by the pink ovoids.

Among the ailments for which Dr William's Pink Pills were claimed to be invaluable were '*Anaemia, Blood Disorders, Bronchitis, Decline, Gastritis, General Weakness, Headache, Indigestion, Influenza's After-Effects, Lumbago, Nervous Debility, Neurasthemia, Neuralgia, Neuritis, Rheumatism, Sciatica, St Vitus' Dance*'. Adverts often consisted of a case study involving the testimonial of a named person with their address followed by a general statement:

Dr William's Pink Pills are in every way as valuable to men as to women, for they possess the unique power of making rich, good blood in abundance; they fill the starved veins with nourishment, so that new energy is carried to every part of the enfeebled system, and in giving this rich, red blood of health they attack the very source of a great number of diseases.

Parents were encouraged to give the pills to their children, especially those who were '*pale, run-down, listless and tire easily*'. The product was highly recommended for girls:

Upon parents rests a great responsibility at the time their daughters are budding into womanhood. If your daughter is pale, complains of weakness, is tired out after the slightest exertion, if she is troubled with headache, backache, if her temper is fitful and her appetite poor, then you may be sure she is a victim of anaemia. In that case you should lose no time in giving your daughter Dr William's Pink Pills. They will assist her to develop properly; they will enrich the blood and restore roses to her cheeks. Wise mothers will give their daughters Dr William's Pink Pills upon the approach of womanhood, and thus avoid the risks of becoming anaemic.

❝ they will enrich the blood and restore roses to her cheeks ❞

Initial analysis of the pills by a Mr George Selkirk — '*an analyst of many years standing*' – specifically for the author of *Exposures to Quackery* in 1895 revealed the presence of '*Extract of Barbadoes Aloes enclosed in a thin coating of sugar, coloured pink with Carmine*', prompting the statement '*we need not look further than these pills for an object lesson on the mean-ness of foisting worthless quack medicines on unfortunate sufferers*'. However, later analyses by the British Medical Association revealed that each pill contained ferrous sulphate, potassium carbonate, magnesia and powdered liquorice and no aloes or arsenic (previously found by an analyst in Australia). The quantities indicated the formula shown here.

Formula, 1905 (amounts after removal of coating)	
Exsiccated sulphate of iron	0.75 grain
Potassium carbonate, anhydrous	0.66 grain
Magnesia	0.09 grain
Powdered liquorice	1.4 grain
Sugar	0.2 grain

Formula, 1935

Iron sulphate	26.66%
Sodium carbonate	26.66%
Powdered aloes	2.66%
Manganese dioxide	1.77%
Zinc phosphid	0.16%
Copper sulphate	0.08%
Extract of gentian	3.33%
Excipients	38.68%

Formula, 1961

Iron sulphate exsiccated	80.99 mg
Copper sulphate	0.65 mg
Manganese sulphate	0.84 mg
Caffeine citrate	32.4 mg
Thiamine hydrochloride	0.156 mg

Over the years this formula has been enhanced and modified several times. In the 1930s the product was declared to contain aloes as well as salts of copper and zinc, presumably to increase its effectiveness as a tonic.

In the 1960s, the formula was radically changed to include caffeine citrate and vitamin B1 (thiamine hydrochloride). The product was withdrawn from the UK market in the 1970s.

Dr William's Medicine Company not only manufactured Dr William's Pills but also Pinklets – a laxative pill – and Bablets – small, soft pellets for teething, cholic and diarrhoea in babies. The company went into receivership in 1989.

Chapter Twenty
Mrs Winslow's Soothing Syrup

*I*n the 1800s it was a commonly held belief by parents, dentists and physicians that teething was one of the *'most perilous transitions'* of childhood being linked to a disease the symptoms of which included sleeplessness, drooling, vomiting, croup, deafness and epilepsy. It is not surprising that, since this developmental stage in children was viewed so seriously, various nostrums based on opiates and morphine were commonplace. One such mixture based on alcohol, morphine in a syrup flavoured with anise was invented in the 1830s by Mrs Charlotte N Winslow, *'an old and experienced nurse'*, from New York who had *'devoted herself for more than thirty years exclusively to the care of children'*. The product was subsequently marketed in a specially moulded slimline bottle embossed with the product name by her son-in-law Jeremiah Curtis and his associate Benjamin Perkins.

Over the next 50 years the popularity of the product climbed to incredible heights and was sold worldwide. Extensive advertising using the full range of marketing techniques available – trade cards, posters, newspaper adverts, endorsements, testimonials, recipe books, almanacs and instructional booklets – assured that the product remained a brand leader. The lithographic images on the trade cards and calendars were in full rich colours, typically portraying an attractive woman dressed in a nightdress or flowing robe either lying on a

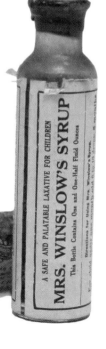

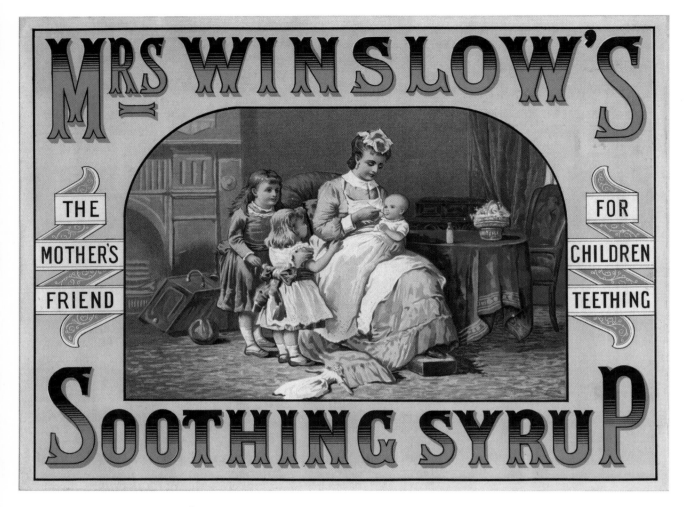

bed or sitting in a parlour, holding or surrounded by one or two healthy, contented children. In all cases the distinctively shaped bottle of Soothing Syrup was positioned either on a nearby nightstand or in the mother's hand, ready for dosing.

In their advice to mothers, Curtis and Perkins claimed:

> the little cherub awakes as bright as a button

MRS WINSLOW'S SOOTHING SYRUP should always be used when children are cutting teeth; it relieves the little sufferer at once, it produces natural quiet sleep by relieving the child from pain, and the little cherub awakes as bright as a button. It is perfectly harmless and very pleasant to taste. It soothes the child, softens the gums, allays all pain and wind, regulates the bowels and is the best known remedy for Dysentery and Diarrhoea, whether arising from teething or other causes.

They also suggested that 'No family should be without a bottle of MRS WINSLOW'S Soothing Syrup in the house. The numerous deaths amongst children might be avoided by its timely use'. This shaming denunciation of women who did not have a bottle of the syrup to hand was also carried in a testimonial in the New York Tribune which stated:

We sincerely believe the mother who has a child suffering from any one of the above complaints (ie teething, dysentery or diarrhoea), and neglects to provide this medicine for its relief and cure, is depriving the little sufferer of the remedy of all in the world best calculated to give it rest and restore it to health.

It is not surprising that with such a potent drug and a popular medicine, babies became comatose or addicted and, on occasions, died. One of the first cases of the latter to be reported was in California in 1869 when a Dr Murray had been called to see a child aged six months, dying from the effects of two teaspoonfuls of Mrs Winslow's Soothing Syrup taken over ten hours. The physician had the mixture analysed and found that it contained 'nearly one grain of morphia and other opium alkaloids to the ounce of syrup'.

Similar cases were reported in San Francisco in 1872. Murray estimated that 100,000 bottles of the syrup were sold annually in California alone. It is interesting to note that the London agents for the product dismissed the analysis as 'absolutely false'. In addition an analysis of the product then sold in the UK was not found to contain any morphine but simply oil of anise. Adverts advised mothers:

If you have a Suffering Child, do not let your prejudices, or the prejudices of others, stand between it and the relief that will be absolutely sure to follow the use of MRS WINSLOW'S SOOTHING SYRUP. It has been used for over 50 years by Millions of Mothers for their children with perfect safety and success.

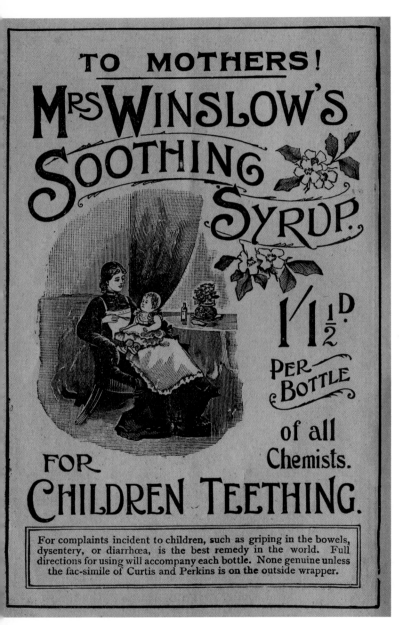

TO MOTHERS!

Mrs WINSLOW'S SOOTHING SYRUP.

1/1½D. PER BOTTLE

of all Chemists.

FOR CHILDREN TEETHING.

For complaints incident to children, such as griping in the bowels, dysentery, or diarrhœa, is the best remedy in the world. Full directions for using will accompany each bottle. None genuine unless the fac-simile of Curtis and Perkins is on the outside wrapper.

Advertisement from *Mrs Winslow's Family Almanac*, 1905 © private collection

Needless to say more deaths were reported in the late 1890s and early 1900s and when the Pure Food and Drug Act became law in the United States on 1 January 1907, Curtis and Perkins were ordered to reduce and then eliminate morphine in their syrup. Between 1908 and 1911 they reduced the amount of morphine in the syrup from 0.4 grain per ounce to 0.16 grain per ounce. In 1915, the US Bureau of Chemistry sued the company. Immediately, before going to court, Curtis and Perkins completely eliminated morphine from the formula and dropped the word 'soothing'. In the UK, prior to 1908 and following cases where unqualified persons were prosecuted for selling the syrup analysed as then containing 0.08 grain of morphine per bottle, the package bore the statement '*this preparation contains, among other valuable ingredients, a small amount of morphine*'. In November 1909, morphine was removed from the product in the UK.

An official analysis of the syrup in 1912 in the UK showed that it contained potassium bromide 2%, alcohol 4.3%, essential oil 0.1% approximately (predominantly oil of anise but which may also have contained a little oil of dill or caraway), sugar 56.5%. Emodin, equivalent to the amount in syrup of senna 1.2%, was also present, as was some evidence of approximately 2% of glycerine. Directions on the label at this time were: '*for a child under one month old, 6–10 drops; three*

MRS. WINSLOW'S
SOOTHING SYRUP
FOR CHILDREN TEETHING.

Greatly facilitates the process of Teething, by softening the Gums, reducing all Inflammation ; will allay ALL PAIN and spasmodic action, and is

SURE TO REGULATE THE BOWELS.

Depend upon it, Mothers, it will give rest to yourselves and

RELIEF & HEALTH TO YOUR INFANTS.

Mrs. WINSLOW'S SOOTHING SYRUP

Has been used for over Fifty Years by millions of Mothers for their children while Teething with perfect success. It soothes the child, softens the gums, allays all pain, cures wind colic, and is the best remedy for diarrhœa.

RETAILED BY CHEMISTS ONLY.

Wholesale from THE ANGLO-AMERICAN DRUG COMPANY (Limited)
33 Farringdon Road, London.

Advertisement reproduced with permission from *The Chemists' and Druggists' Diary*, 1900

months old, half a teaspoonful; six months old and upwards, a teaspoonful three or four times a day. For Dysentery, repeat the above dose every two hours, until the character of the discharges is changed for the better'.

Over the next two decades the formulation was modified further, both potassium bromide and alcohol being eliminated in favour of sodium citrate and sodium bicarbonate. In the mid 1930s Curtis and Perkins ceased manufacturing the product in the USA. In the UK production was continued by Thos Christy and Company Ltd, based in Aldershot. In 1943 claims for the product were modified to: '*A stomach and bowel regulator for infants and children. For children teething. A safe remedy for digestive troubles, constipation and diarrhea, feverishness and restlessness*', in line with the ingredients used. The product continued to be sold in the UK in this guise until it was withdrawn in the early 1960s.

Formula, 1940s (in UK)

Sodium citrate	2.160%
Oil of anise	0.059%
Extract of rhubarb	0.040%
Oil of coriander	0.012%
Extract of senna	0.236%
Oil of fennel	0.069%
Sodium bicarbonate	0.223%
Oil of caraway	0.040%
Sucrose	61.339%
Distilled water	35.802%

WOODWARD'S "GRIPE WATER"

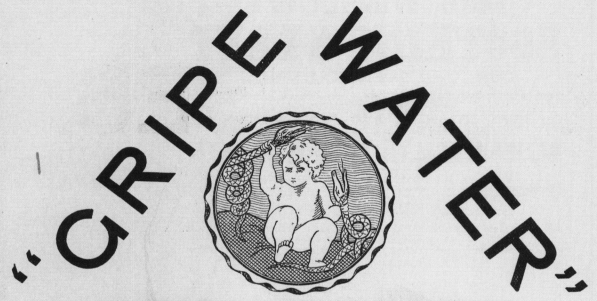

FOR ALL DISORDERS OF INFANTS AND YOUNG CHILDREN.

For Wholesale and Export terms apply

W. WOODWARD, CHAUCER STREET, NOTTINGHAM.

FOREIGN AND COLONIAL AGENTS.

AFRICA.

CAPE COLONY:

ALIWAL NORTH	Messrs. Lennon & Co.
BEAUFORT WEST	,, ,, ,,
CAPE TOWN ...	,, Heynes, Mathew & Co.
,, ,, ...	,, Lennon & Co.
,, ,, ...	,, Peterson & Co.
,, ,, ...	,, Pocock & Co.
,, ,, ...	,, Sainsbury & Co.
EAST LONDON .	,, Lennon & Co.
GRAAF REINET	,, ,,
KIMBERLEY......	,, ,,
OUDTSHOORN ...	,, ,,
PAARL	,, ,,
PORT ELIZA-BETH.........}	,, Gardner & Co.
,, ,,	,, Lennon & Co.
,, ,,	,, Willett & Co.

NATAL:

DURBAN.........	Mr. H. J. Brereton.
,, ...	The Natal Drug Co. (Lim.)
PIETERMARITZ-BURG ....}	Messrs. Stantiel & Allerston.
,,	Turner & Co.

AFRICA—(continued).

ORANGE RIVER COLONY:

BLOEMFONTEIN...	Messrs. Lennon & Co.
WYNBERG	,, ,,

RHODESIA:

BULUWAYO	Messrs. Lennon & Co.

TRANSVAAL:

FORDSBURG	Messrs. Corry & Co.
,, ...	,, Lennon & Co.
JOHANNESBURG...	,, ,,
,, ...	,, Loewenstein & Co.
,, ...	,, Peterson & Co.
,, ...	,, Turner & Co.
NEW PRIMROSE...	,, Corry & Co.
PRETORIA	,, Phillips & Co.

AMERICA.

NEW YORK	Messrs. Fougera & Co.
PATERSON, N.J....	Mr. C. P. Kinsilla.

AUSTRALIA.

NEW SOUTH WALES:

SYDNEY	Messrs. Sayers, Allport & Potter.

QUEENSLAND:

BRISBANE	Messrs. Taylor & Colledge.

SOUTH AUSTRALIA:

ADELAIDE	Messrs. J. F. Faulding & Co.

VICTORIA:

MELBOURNE ...	Messrs. Duerdin & Sainsbury.

WEST AUSTRALIA:

PERTH............	Messrs. J. F. Faulding & Co.

NEW ZEALAND:

AUCKLAND	Messrs. Sharland & Co. (Lim.).
WELLINGTON ...	,, ,,

INDIA.

CALCUTTA	Messrs. Smith, Stanistreet & Co.
	Messrs. Bathgate & Co.
MADRAS	,, Smith & Co.

Chapter Twenty-one
Woodward's Gripe Water

*T*he man who gave his name to Woodward's Gripe Water was born in Stamford, Lincolnshire, in 1828. Having attended Stamford Grammar School, William Woodward, aged 14, was apprenticed to John Holliday Thomas, a pharmacist in Boston, Lincolnshire, 34 miles away. At the end of his seven years' apprenticeship, Woodward moved to London, and got a job in Fetter Lane, just off Fleet Street. He stayed in London for a year. Woodward moved out to Nottingham in 1851 and bought his own pharmacy in the Market Place. An article in *The Chemist and Druggist* in 1914 stated '*Mr Woodward was gifted with a scientific mind, and soon established for himself a reputation as a technical adviser in respect to all matters dealing with local industries*'.

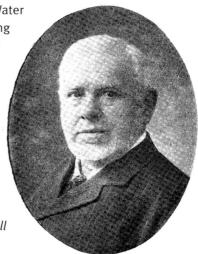

THE LATE WILLIAM WOODWARD.

Woodward developed his gripe water to give babies relief from colic, wind and indigestion, soon after he moved to Nottingham. He sold it by the ounce to customers, and by the gallon to medical practitioners, hospitals and wholesale houses. It seems that its reputation grew without any proactive advertising by Woodward. Woodward registered the description 'Gripe Water' as a trademark in 1876, on the grounds that it had been in use for 25 years prior to the date of application. At the same time, Woodward also registered an engraving of Sir Joshua Reynolds's painting *The Infant Hercules* as a trademark, for use on his bottle labels.

Above: Reproduced with permission from *The Chemist + Druggist Magazine*, 1914

Left: Advertisement reproduced with permission from *The Chemists' and Druggists' Diary*, 1902

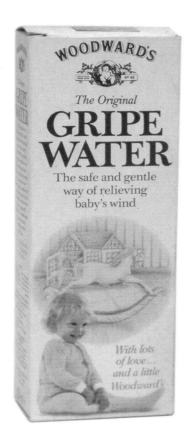

Woodward retired from his pharmacy in 1877. However, rather than including his gripe water in the sale of his business, he asked his friend Richard Fitzhugh, a justice of the peace and pharmaceutical chemist, to take it over. Apparently bored in retirement, Woodward bought the gripe water business back five years later. He built premises at Chaucer Street in Nottingham to make and distribute the product.

In May 1903, a limited company was registered to take over from Mr Woodward, with the recipes for Gripe Water and other products, and to carry on the business. Woodward was the permanent governing director until his death at his home in London on 1 September 1912, aged 85.

The founder's son, William Harrison Woodward, had been involved in the running of the business for about 10 years before his father's death. WH Woodward was a writer, lecturer and founder of a training college affiliated with the University of Liverpool. Although he became governing director on his father's death, WH Woodward continued with his literary pursuits, and spent part of each year in Italy.

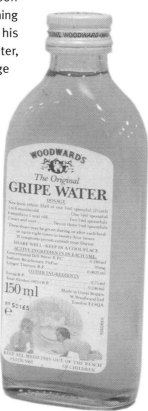

In 1913, John C Umney became joint managing director of the company with WH Woodward. In 1914, an article in *The Chemist and Druggist* gave a detailed description of the company and its premises: '*one part of the factory was steam and compounding laboratories, other parts were used for bottle-washing and bottle-filling, and a whole floor was used for packing. The administrative offices were also on the same site*'.

In the same year, Gripe Water was placed on the list of the Proprietary Articles Trade Association.

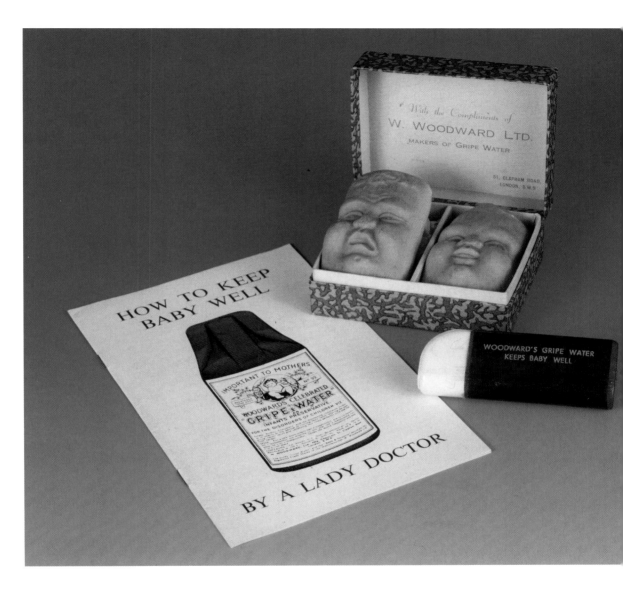

This coincided with a significant increase in global advertising for the product, and a renewed assertion of the company's exclusive right to the trademark Gripe Water. *The Chemist and Druggist* (31 January 1914, page 153) stated that there is '*quite a respectable sale for the Gripe Water in China, where a penny has not been spent on advertising it; in fact, the popularity is chiefly due to the ladies of the American and European legations using it for their children and recommending it to their friends*'. The same article explained that a question to the company

Promotional items including 'happy' and 'sad' baby face soaps © Royal Pharmaceutical Society

about the stability of the product in a tropical climate received the response that there had never been a complaint received on this matter. At its height, Gripe Water became renowned in over 50 countries globally, often introduced by the wives of serving army personnel. In 1969, company publicity stated that the product was being made locally in Canada, South Africa, Australia, India, Pakistan and Ghana.

The factory moved to Tufnell Park, North London in 1920. One half of the company's capital was acquired by The Sanitas Company Ltd in 1923. In 1926, on the formation of the Sanitas Trust Ltd, the remaining shareholding was bought out from Levers by the trust. At the same time, the manufacture of Woodward's Gripe Water was transferred to Sanitas's Limehouse factory. The company acquired Oppenheimer, and at this stage the manufacture of the Gripe Water was transferred to Clapham Road. Gripe Water was the company's sole product, described in October 1969 as '*a celebrated carminative for the relief of babies' minor tummy ailments*'.

> **" a celebrated carminative for the relief of babies' minor tummy ailments "**

The formula was reputedly based on an original recipe discovered by a small group of Nottingham doctors, to treat what was known locally as 'fen fever'. The bottle's label said:

Woodward's Celebrated Gripe Water, or Infant's Preservative, without Laudanum, for all disorders of children, viz.: Convulsions, Gripes, Acidity, Flatulency, Whooping-Cough, and the distressing complaints incidental to Infants at the period of Cutting their Teeth, allaying the pain, giving instant relief, and rendering this crisis perfectly mild and free from danger.

Formula, 1909

Analysis (100 parts by measure)	
Sodium bicarbonate	1.08 part
Essential oil	about 0.03 part
Alcohol	3.8 parts by measure
Sugar	20.5 parts

Secret Remedies described it as a carminative water containing less than 4% alcohol. No alkaloid was present, and the essential oil was identified as primarily oil of caraway, with a little oil of dill, and possibly some oil of anise. The recommended dose for an infant was half a teaspoonful, increasing to one or two teaspoonfuls for a two-month-old child.

The presence of alcohol in a preparation intended for

infants created the potential for controversy. At an inquiry of a government select committee on proprietary medicines in 1913, John Umney gave evidence to the committee stating that the analysis in *Secret Remedies* was wrong. He claimed that the analysis had both missed the most important ingredient and detected substances in the Gripe Water that were never there. Nevertheless, the Principal Government Chemist had testified that the preparation contained less than 4% alcohol. Umney explained that the alcohol was necessary as a solvent, and that '*we have tried dozens of ways to avoid alcohol*' but that it was necessary. He explained that the company would be keen to obtain the same therapeutic effect another way. At the same inquiry, Umney was questioned about paying people to provide testimonials. He denied that this was the case, but admitted that the company had given a man 72 bottles of the gripe water in return for printing his testimonial. Umney refused to admit that this was remuneration for the testimonial itself, but for its publication.

By 1972, Gripe Water had been joined by other Woodward's products – baby cream and baby wipes. In the 34th edition of *Martindale*, published in 2005, Woodward's Gripe Water containing terpeneless dill seed oil and sodium bicarbonate is included. The product was being made by Pharmacare in Canada, LRC in Israel and SSL in the UK. Other Woodward's products given are Baby Chest Rub, Colic Drops, Diaper Rash, Inhalant, Nappy Rash Ointment and Teething Gel, although only the Rub, Colic Drops, Gripe Water and Nappy Rash Ointment are produced in the UK.

Formula, 1972	
Dill water concentrated	3.6%
Sodium bicarbonate	1%
Ginger tincture	1.25%
Rectified spirit	3.67%
Syrup	22.5%

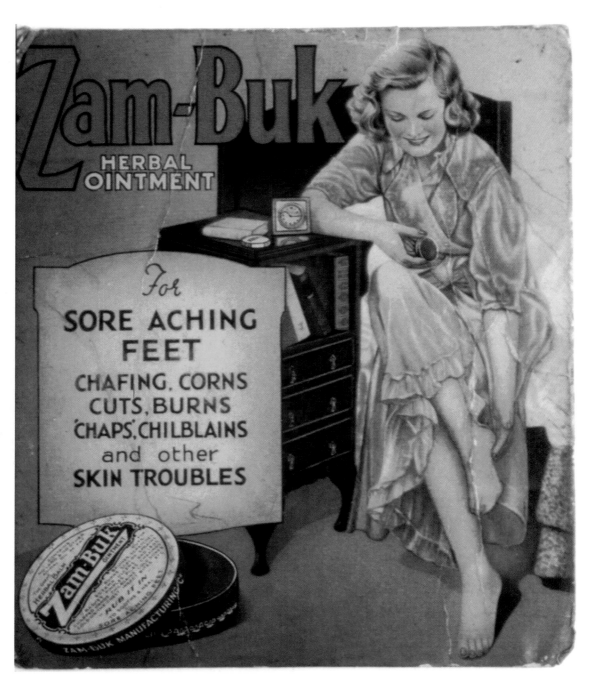

Chapter Twenty-two
Zam-Buk

Bile Beans were not Charles Fulford's only success. In 1903 he introduced Zam-Buk ointment, which he claimed had been successfully used by a former officer in the Indian Medical Service. In a circular enclosed with the product it was related how:

certain medicinal plants were taken, and from them were extracted gums and juices possessing considerable healing and curative power. Costly experiments at last secured the right blending of these juices; and to the final product, a preparation virtually capable of growing new and healthy skin, the name of Zam-Buk was given. Zam-Buk practically contains those substances which Nature has intended for the use of man ever since she bequeathed to him the instinct to rub a place that hurts.

Zam-Buk was widely advertised for a whole variety of complaints including:

Cuts, Bruises, Burns, Scalds, Abrasions, Festering Sores, Poisoned Wounds, Lacerated Wounds, Old Wounds, Sprains, Strains, Swellings, Dog Bites, Cat Scratches, Obstinate Sores, Chafings, Itch (Scabies), Stings from Hornets, Bees, Wasps, Centipedes, and

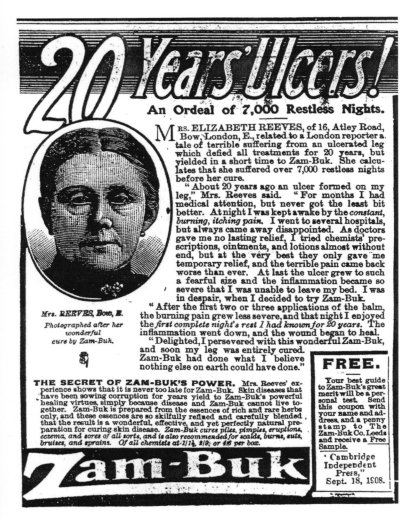

THE SECRET OF ZAM-BUK'S POWER. Mrs. Reeves' experience shows that it is never too late for Zam-Buk. Skin diseases that have been sowing corruption for years yield to Zam-Buk's powerful healing virtues, simply because disease and Zam-Buk cannot live together. Zam-Buk is prepared from the essences of rich and rare herbs only, and these essences are so skilfully refined and carefully blended, that the result is a wonderful, effective, and yet perfectly natural preparation for curing skin disease. Zam-Buk cures piles, pimples, eruptions, eczema, and sores of all sorts, and is also recommended for scalds, burns, cuts, bruises, and sprains. Of all chemists at 1/1½, 2/9, or 4/6 per box.

Spiders; Running Sores, Ulcers, Ringworm, Eczema (acute or chronic form), Psoriasis (tetter), Pimples, Acne, Abscesses, Boils, Carbuncles, Scrofula, Cramp, Barber's Itch, Heat Rashes, Sunburn, Freckles, Blotches, Blackheads, Scalp Irritations, Scurf or Dandruff, and other Scalp Sores; Colds, Chills, Raw Chapped Hands, Sore Lips, Raw Chin after Shaving; Inflamed Patches, Sore Nipples, Glandular Swellings, Swollen Knees, Bad Legs, Blind and Bleeding Piles, Cold-Sores, Sore Backs, Diseased or Weak Ankles, Sore and Aching Feet, Perspiring Feet, Chilblains, Soft Corns and Saltwater Sores. Rubbed well into the part affected, Zam-Buk gives great relief from Rheumatism, Lumbago, Neuralgia, Sciatica, Toothache, and all kinds of Inflammation, Itching and Irritation.

Again, as with Bile Beans, extensive advertising and endorsements ensured that Zam-Buk soon became a household name and a very successful product. An advert in the *Cambridge Independent Press* dated 18 September 1908 was typical of those produced at this time.

It relates how a Mrs Elizabeth Reeves from London had suffered for 20 years with an ulcerated leg until, in desperation, she had tried Zam-Buk. After the first two or three applications of the balm, the inflammation went down and the wound began to heal. The postscript under the heading *The Secret of Zam-Buk's Power* states:

Mrs Reeves experience shows that it is never too late for Zam-Buk. Skin diseases that have been sowing corruption for years yield to Zam-Buk's powerful healing virtues, simply because disease and Zam-Buk cannot live together. Zam-Buk is prepared from the essences of rich and rare herbs only, and these essences are so skilfully refined and carefully blended that the result is a wonderful, effective, and yet perfectly natural preparation for curing skin disease.

Other adverts at this time refer to Zam-Buk being '*made like the rich balms used by the gladiators of Ancient Greece*' and in the case of ringworm and eczema in children '*Zam-Buk soaks right through the diseased tissue and kills the microscopic fungus plants and parasites which are the cause of the trouble, afterwards restoring the scalp and skin to sweetness and health*'. A Zam-Buk march was even composed and the music for the piano was published in 1907.

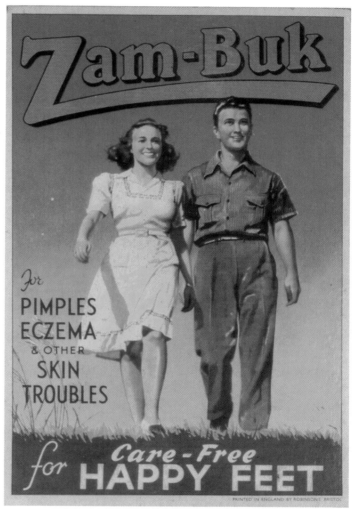

© Museum of Brands

In all adverts, much was made of the '*natural, pure saps, juices and aromatic oils from healing herbs*' used in the preparation of the product unlike '*ordinary preparations which contain quantities of animal fat and mineral poisons, and are coarse, risky and unreliable.*' However, a detailed analysis in 1909 showed it to simply contain oil of eucalyptus 14%, colophony 20%, soft paraffin 55%, hard paraffin 11% and a trace of green colouring matter, possibly chlorophyll. The estimated cost of the ingredients was only 2% of the selling price.

The product was packaged in a round tin and manufactured by the Zam-Buk Manufacturing Company part of CE Fulford Ltd, Leeds, UK. The

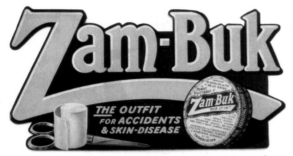

© Museum of Brands

" In our opinion it would add greatly to the efficiency of the Army "

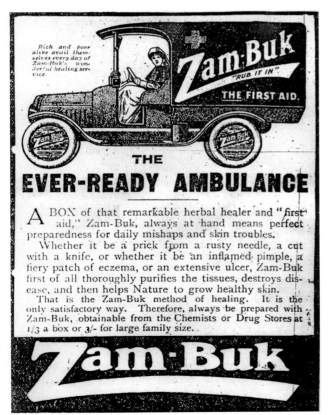

© private collection

company then had branches and agencies throughout the world especially in Australia (Sydney, Adelaide, Melbourne, Brisbane, Perth) South Africa (Cape Town), Tasmania (Launceston), New Zealand (Dunedin, Auckland), Canada (Toronto) and India (Calcutta).

During the First World War, Zam-Buk was openly advertised for use by soldiers and sailors to heal cuts, bad feet and trench sores. It was stated that soldiers and sailors preferred Zam-Buk because of '*its unique curative properties, its compact and concentrated character which results in more soothing, healing and antiseptic power being contained in a box of Zam-Buk than can be found in twenty times the same bulk of other ointments, and its unfailing reliability*'. In one advert the War Office was quoted as saying '*We should like to see a box or two of this excellent "first-aid", Zam-Buk, supplied to every soldier. In our opinion it would add greatly to the efficiency of the Army*'. In 1918 the product was advertised as the '*The Ever-Ready Ambulance*' with a nurse driving an ambulance with tins of Zam-Buk for wheels. It may well be at this time that the product name first became a nickname for members of the St John Ambulance Brigade.

The product remained a brand leader throughout the 1920s, 1930s and 1940s. In 1931 it was claimed as being '*the most universally sold proprietary skin ointment in the world*'. Trade adverts in 1939 stressed the popularity of the ointment in the home, at work and on the sports ground. In addi-

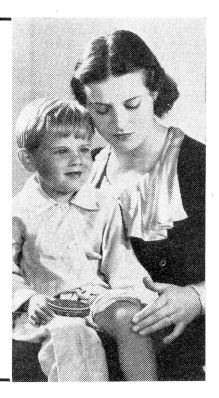

EVERY HOME NEEDS

Zam-Buk

Brand Ointment

There's always a good steady sale for Zam-Buk, which for over thirty-five years has been the most popular skin ointment in the home, at work and on the sports ground. Zam-Buk is useful all the year round, so don't let your stock get low.

ZAM-BUK MEDICINAL SOAP

Specially recommended for tender skins, as a shampoo and for use with Zam-Buk Ointment in skin trouble.

ZAM-BUK SUPPOSITORIES

Zam-Buk Ointment in soluble Suppository form. A very popular and succesful treatment for inward piles.

Sole Proprietors: C. E. FULFORD, LTD., LEEDS

tion the company supplied the product in the form of a medicinal soap for bathing and suppositories for piles. By this time the formulation had changed somewhat with the addition of camphor, oil of thyme and sassafras oil.

In the 1950s the sassafras oil was removed and slight changes were made in the proportions of the other ingredients but the tin remained the same.

In 1964 the company was acquired by Fisons Ltd, Loughborough, for £1.1 million. Zam-Buk continued to be manufactured by Fisons until 1993 when it was divested to Roche. Roche Consumer UK continued to market the product in the UK until the mid-1990s when it was withdrawn from sale. However, Roche continue to manufacture and market the product containing sassafras oil in South Africa for wounds, burns, pruritus, chapped hands, insect bites and

Advertisement from Butler and Crispe catalogue, 1939
© Royal Pharmaceutical Society

Formula, 1935	
Resin Pini Palust. (colophony)	14.40%
Paraffin Dur. (hard paraffin)	21.50%
Paraffin Molle (soft paraffin)	53.40%
Ol Eucalypt. Globul. (Eucalyptus oil)	7.56%
Flor. Camphorae (Flowers of camphor)	1.85%
Ol Thyme Vulgar. (Wild thyme oil)	0.93%
Ext. Chlorophylli. (Chlorophyll)	0.03%
Ol Sassaf. Officin. (Sassafrax oil)	0.33%

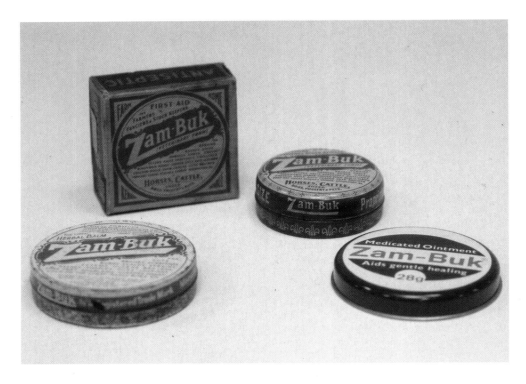

muscular pain. In Australia the product was, until recently, marketed by Key Phamaceuticals and was sold in tubes.

Although Zam-Buk may have vanished from the shelves of pharmacies in the UK, it is still available from Feathergills of Hebden Bridge, West Yorkshire, UK. It is interesting to note that the ointment is still packaged in a round tin with a label not unlike the original first marketed over a century ago. The indications include *'cuts, bruises, burns, scalds, sprains, eczema, ulcers, chapped hands, sores, insect bites, chilblains, rashes, rheumatism, cold sores etc.'*.

Further Reading

Journals

The Pharmaceutical Journal, 1841–

The Chemist and Druggist, 1860–

The Lancet, 1823–

The Pharmaceutical Historian, 1967–

Pharmacy in History, 1959–

General books

Beasley H. *Pocket Formulary*, 2nd edn 1842; 12th edn 1899. London: Churchill.

British Medical Association and Royal Pharmaceutical Society of Great Britain. *British National Formulary*, 1st edn 1957-–present. London: BMA and RPSGB.

Pharmaceutical Formulas. 1st edn 1898–11th edn 1956. London: *The Chemist and Druggist*.

The Chemists' and Druggists' Diary 1886–1934.

The Chemists' and Druggists' Diary and Yearbook 1935–1968

The Chemist and Druggist Yearbook and Buyer's Guide 1969

The Chemist and Druggist Yearbook 1970–1971.

The Chemist and Druggist Directory 1972–present.

Editor, *Health News* (1895). *Exposures of Quackery*, vols I and 2. London: Savoy Press.

Holloway SWF (1991). *Royal Pharmaceutical Society of Great Britain 1841–1991. A political and social history*. London: Pharmaceutical Press.

British Medical Association (1909). *Secret Remedies: what they cost and what they contain*. London: BMA.

British Medical Association (1912). *More Secret Remedies: what they cost and what they contain*. London: BMA.

Squire P. *Squire's Pocket Book Companion to the British Pharmacopoeia*. 1st edn 1864–19th edn 1916. London: Whittaker.

Thompson CJS (1928). *The Quacks of Old London*. London: Brentano's Ltd.

Martindale: The Extra Pharmacopoeia, 1st edn 1883 – present. London: Pharmaceutical Press.

Specific medicines

Chapter 2 – Anderson's Scots Pills

Jackson WA (1987). Grana Angelica: Patrick Anderson and the True Scots Pills. *Pharmaceutical Historian* 17: 2–5.

Comrie JD (1932). *History of Scottish Medicine*. London: Balliere, Tyndall & Cox.

Chapter 3 – Beecham's Pills

Anderson SC, Homan PG (2002). Best for me, best for you – a history of Beecham's Pills 1842–1998. *Pharmaceutical Journal* 269: 921–924.

Francis A (1986). *A Guinea a Box*. London: Robert Hale.

Lazell HG (1975). *From Pills to Penicillin: the Beecham Story*. London: Heinemann.

Chapter 4 – Bile Beans

Rowe RC (2003). Bile Beans for Inner Health. *International Journal of Pharmaceutical Medicine* 17: 137–140.

Chapter 5 – Burgess's Lion ointment

Lion Ointment. *Chemist and Druggist* 3 Jan 1976, 16–17.

Chapter 10 – Fennings' Children's Cooling Powders

Formulae for success. *Wholesale Grocer* Mar 1984, 43.

Chapter 11 – Holloway's Pills and Ointment

Harrison-Barbet A (1990). *Thomas Holloway: Victorian Philanthropist. A biographical essay*. Egham, Surrey: Royal Holloway College.

Chapter 12 – Dr James's Fever Powders

Cox TM, Jack N, Lofthouse S, *et al.* (2005). King George III and porphyria: an elemental hypothesis and investigation. *Lancet* 366: 332–335.

Bishop TH (1955). 250 years ago was born Robert James M.D. of "fever powder" fame. *Chemist and Druggist* 22 Jan: 94.

Corley TAB (1987). Interactions between the British and American Patent Medicine Industries 1708–1914. In: Atack J, ed. *Business and Economic History*, 2nd series, vol. 16. Chicago, Illinois: University of Illinois.

Crellin JK (1974). Dr James's Fever Powder. *Transactions of the British Society of History of Pharmacy* 1: 136–143.

Donovan M (1869). On the Process for Preparing James's Powder. *Pharmaceutical Journal* 11: 142.

Pulvis Jacobi Verus and Other Old Medicines. *Chemist and Druggist* 25 Jul 1896, 160–161.

Chapter 13 – Morison's Pills

Morison J (1831). *Morisonia*. London.

Helfand William H (1974). James Morison and his pills. A study of the nineteenth century pharmaceutical market. *Transactions of the British Society for the History of Pharmacy* 1: 3.

Chapter 14 – Mother Seigel's Syrup

Corley TAB (1987). Interactions between the British and American Patent Medicine Industries 1708–1914. In: Atack J, ed. *Business and Economic History*, 2nd series, vol. 16. Chicago, Illinois: University of Illinois.

Mother Seigel on her Travels. *Chemist and Druggist* 15 Oct 1880, 448.

Chapter 15 – Lydia E Pinkham's Vegetable Compound

Jackson WA (1998). Who Was Lily the Pink? *Pharmaceutical Historian* 28 (July): 22–28.

Stage S (1979). *Female Complaints: Lydia Pinkham and the business of women's medicine.* New York: WW Norton.

Varro ET (1995). Was Lydia E Pinkham's Vegetable Compound an effective remedy? *Pharmaceutical Historian* 37: 24–28.

Chapter 16 – Poor Man's Friend Ointment

Bridport Town's Coffee Tavern. *Chemist and Druggist*, 29 Aug 1959, 125–127.

Chapter 18 – Steedman's Soothing Powders

John Steedman & Co., Walworth. 127 Years of Pharmaceutical Control. *Pharmaceutical Journal* 18 Nov 1939, 444–445.

Proprietary Medicines Inquiry. Proceedings Before Select Committee. *Pharmaceutical Journal* 15 Feb 1913, 214–215.

Chapter 19 – Dr William's Pink Pills for Pale People

Loeb L (1999). George Fulford and Victorian Patent Medicine; Quack Mercenaries or Smilesian Entrepreneurs? *Canadian Bulletin of Medical History* 16: 125–145.

Miller G (2001). Pills for Pale People; The George Fulford Story. *Pharmacy History Australia* 13 (March): 3–5.

Chapter 20 – Mrs Winslow's Soothing Syrup

McNutt WF (1872). Mrs Winslow's Soothing Syrup – A Poison. *American Journal of Pharmacy* 1 May: 221–224.

Christen AG, Christen JA (2000). Sozodont Powder Dentifrice and Mrs Winslow's Soothing Syrup: Dental Nostrums. *Journal of the History of Dentistry* 48: 99–105.

Chapter 21 – Woodward's Gripe Water

Gripe-water. *Chemist and Druggist*, 31 January 1914, 152–154.

Proprietary Medicines Inquiry. Proceedings Before Select Committee. *Pharmaceutical Journal* 15 Feb 1913, 214–215.

Chapter 22 – Zam Buk

Howie-Willis I (2001). Who or What is Zam buk? *Pharmacy History Australia* 15 (Nov): 6–8.

Glossary

Alterative	A medicine that alters the processes of nutrition and excretion, restoring normal body functions
Anodyne	A medicine for relieving pain
Antispasmodic	Counteraction to spasms of the stomach
Aperient	Laxative
Aromatic	Spicy and fragrant
Astringent	An agent producing contraction of organic tissues or the arrest of a discharge
Bitter	Appetite stimulant
Bloody flux	Dysentery
Carminative	A medicine expelling flatus
Cathartic	A laxative medicine
Cholagogue	Promotes the flow of bile
Consumption	Tuberculosis
Costiveness	Constipation
Decline	Wasting away
Decoction	An extract of plant ingredient that is soluble in water
Demulcent	A mucilaginous substance to allay irritation (in coughs, etc.)
Diaphoretic	Produces perspiration
Diuretic	Increases the flow of urine
Dropsy	Fluid in the tissues and cavities of the body
Emetic	Induces vomiting
Emmenagogue	Stimulates menstrual flow
Excipient	A substance added to a drug to aid formulation and assist in the manufacture of a medicine
Expectorant	Promotes the secretion of bronchial mucus

Exsiccated	Dried
Ext.	Extract: a fluid or solid concentration of plant matter by soaking in alcohol or water then evaporating off excess liquor
Febrile	Pertaining to fever
Fluid Extract	See Ext.
Gravel	Sand-like deposits in the bladder
Green sickness	Chlorosis –- a form of anaemia giving a greenish colour to the skin
Hepatic stimulant	Stimulates liver action
Hooping-cough	Whooping cough
Hydrophobia	Rabies
Megrim	Migraine
Neurasthenia	Exhaustion of the nerve force
Palsy	Paralysis
Purgative	Produces watery evacuations
q.s.	Quantum sufficiat (sufficient quantity)
Quinsy	Severe inflammation of the tonsils with fever
Res.	Resin
Scorbutic	Pertaining to scurvy
Scrofula	Tuberculosis of the glands. Also known as the King's Evil
Scurvy	Illness due to lack of Vitamin C
Sedative	Soothing; allays irritation
Soporific	Produces sleep
Stimulant	Quickening or increasing a body function
Stomachic	A stomach stimulant
Sudorific	Induces sweating
Tincture	Alcoholic extract of plants
Tonic	Agent promoting the normal tone of an organ
Vermifuge	Agent to expel intestinal worms
v/v	Volume in volume
v/w	Volume in weight
w/v	Weight in volume
w/w	Weight in weight

Substances Used in Remedies

Substances mentioned in the book are described below. The uses of the substances stated are concurrent with the beliefs at the time of the remedy and do not necessarily relate to usage in modern medicine.

Actaea racemosa	*see* Cimicifuga
Aletris farinosa	Also known as unicorn root. A so-called uterine tonic
Algaroth powder	A mixed variety of types of antimony
Alkaloid	An active ingredient extracted from a plant, eg morphine from opium
Aloes	A laxative
Aloes Barb.	Aloes from Barbados
Anise	Aniseed flavour and carminative
Aniseed oil	As Anise
Antimony	Diaphoretic, expectorant and emetic
Asafoetida	Also known as Devil's Dung. A nerve stimulant, expectorant and carminative
Asclepias tuberosa	*see* Pleurisy root
Bismuth oxide	Used as an anti-itch ingredient in ointments
Black cohosh	*see* Cimicifuga
Black hellebore	Purgative and emmenagogue
Bromvaleton	A sedative and mild hypnotic
Buckthorn	*Rhamnus cathartica*. A purgative
Caffeine citrate	Nerve stimulant
Calc. Phosph.	Calcium for nutrition and antacid
Calcium carbonate	Antacid
Calomel	Alterative, purgative and anti-syphilitic
Cambogia	*see* Gamboge

Capsicine	The main ingredient of the capsicum
Capsicum	Hot American pepper
Caraway	Flavour and carminative
Carbonate of magnesia	Antacid and mild laxative
Cardam.	*see* Cardamom
Cardamom	Flavour and carminative
Cascara	Laxative
Cascarin	An ingredient of Cascara
Castor	Dried secretions from the beaver. Stimulant and antispasmodic. Treatment of dysmenorrhoea
Chamomile	Tonic, aromatic and stomachic
Chimafila	*Chimaphila*. Diuretic
Chloric Ether	1 part of chloroform in 20 parts of alcohol. Also known as Spirit of Chloroform
Chloroform	Anaesthetic. Used internally as an antispasmodic and a sedative for asthma, colic, cough and neuralgia
Chlorophylli	Green colouring of plants
Cimicifuga	*Actaea racemosa* or Black cohosh. Used for rheumatism and amenorrhoea
Codeine	An ingredient of opium. Relieves pain, diarrhoea and coughs
Colocynth	Very strong laxative
Colophony	Rosin. Applied to wounds to stop bleeding
Copper sulphate	Emetic, tonic and astringent
Coriander	Flavour and carminative
Cream of tartar	Diuretic and cathartic
Crocus	*see* Saffron
Dandelion	Mildly laxative bitter
Dill	Flavour and carminative
Ether	Anaesthetic and solvent
Eucalyptus	Antiseptic and aromatic for colds and catarrh
Euonymus atropurpureus	Tonic, laxative and diuretic
Fennel	Flavour and carminative
Flor. Camphorae	Flowers of camphor

Foenugreek	Was used for diabetes and fever
Gamboge	A vermifuge
Gaultheria procumbens	*see* Wintergreen
Gentian	A bitter tonic
Gentiana rubra	*see* Gentian
Ginger	Used for nausea and vomiting, arthritis and menstrual cramps
Glycyrrh.	*see* Liquorice
Glycyrrhiza	*see* Liquorice
Gum ammoniacum	Expectorant
Hard soap	A binding agent in the making of pills
Heavy magnesium carbonate	Antacid
Hydrastis canadensis	Used internally as a bitter tonic, and for intermittent fevers, menorrhagia and dysmenorrhoea and gonorrhoea. Used externally for ulcers and acne
Hydrochloric acid	Used to treat indigestion caused by lack of stomach acid
Hydrocyanic acid	Used in painful dyspepsia and to allay vomiting and cough
Indian hemp	Pain and insomnia
Ipecacuanha	Expectorant and emetic
Ipomoeia	Laxative
Iris versicolor	Laxative
Iron sulphate	Tonic
Jalap	Strong laxative
Juglans regia	Hepatic stimulant and laxative
Kaolin	Absorbent, treatment of diarrhoea
Lactos.	Lactose – milk sugar
Lard	Animal fat used as an ointment base
Laudanum	Tincture of opium (*see* Opium)
Lead oleate	Used in adhesive plaster
Leptandra	Also known as black root laxative
Leptandrin	Extract of Leptandra
Life root	*Senecio aureus*. Uterine tonic, diuretic and laxative
Light kaolin	*see* Kaolin
Light magnesium carbonate	Antacid and mild laxative

Light magnesium oxide	Antacid and mild laxative
Lignum sassafras	Used externally as an antifungal and against body lice
Liquorice	Demulcent, flavouring and sweetening
Mag. Carb. Lev.	Antacid and mild laxative
Mag. Oxid. Pond	Antacid and mild laxative
Manganese dioxide	Tonic and alterative
Manganese sulphate	Tonic and cathartic
Mercuric oxide	Used externally as an antiseptic
Mercury subchloride	*see* Calomel
Morphia	*see* Morphine
Morphine	A main constituent of opium for coughs, pain, sedation and diarrhoea
Myrrh	A stimulant tonic
Nitric acid dilute	Tonic, promotes bile
Nutmeg oil	Flavour and carminative
Ol Eucalypt. Globul.	Eucalyptus oil. Fragrant and antispasmodic
Ol. Sassaf. Officin.	Sassafras oil. Used for rheumatism and skin problems
Ol. Thyme Vulgar	Wild thyme oil. Used in whooping cough and bronchitis
Olive oil	Used in making ointments and liniments and internally as a mild laxative and enema
Opium	Pain relief, coughs and diarrhoea
Orris	Laxative and diuretic. Used in dropsy
Paracetamol	Pain relief
Pennyroyal	Emmenagogue, irritant to the kidneys and bladder
Pepper	Carminative and diuretic
Peppermint oil	Stomach sedative, aids digestion
Perchloric acid	*see* Hydrochloric acid
Phenacet.	Phenacetin — for pain
Phenolphthalein	Purgative
Phytolacca	Also known as poke root emetic, purgative and used for chronic rheumatism
Pleurisy root	Expectorant and diuretic
Podoph.	Podophyllum. Cholagogue and aperient

Pot. Chloras	Potassium chlorate. Used for inflammation of the mouth
Potassium bromide	A sedative
Potassium carbonate	Antacid
Proof spirit	Alcohol approximately 51% v/v
Prussic acid	*see* Hydrocyanic acid
Quinine	Used against fevers and malaria, and as a tonic
Rectified spirit	Pure alcohol
Resin Piny Palust.	*see* Colophony
Rhubarb	Laxative and astringent
Rosin	*see* Colophony
Saffron	Emmenagogue and used to treat measles
Sapo dura	Hard soap
Saponis Cast.	Castile soap
Sassafras	Carminative
Scammon.	Scammony. A powerful laxative
Senecio aureus	*see* Life root
Senna	Laxative
Sodium bicarbonate	Antacid. Once used in diabetes
Sodium carbonate	Internal antiseptic
Sodium citrate	Diaphoretic, diuretic. Used in the treatment of cystitis
Sodium tauroglycocholate	Cholagogue. Assists pancreatic digestion
Spermaceti	Wax obtained from whales and used in ointments
Starch	A bulking agent in pills, powders and tablets
Stillingia	Queen's root. Used for syphilis, jaundice and piles
Stillingia officinalis	As Stillingia
Sugar of lead	Lead acetate. Used internally to treat severe diarrhoea and bleeding stomach ulcers. Used externally for bruises, eczema and itching
Sulphate of soda	Sodium sulphate or Glauber salts – a laxative
Taraxacum officinale	*see* Dandelion
Turpentine	Carminative, expectorant and diuretic. Used in cystitis and against intestinal worms. Used externally for rheumatism and stiffness
Unicorn root	*see Aletris farinosa*

Venetian red	Ferric oxide. Red colouring matter
Venetian turpentine	Used externally for rheumatism and stiffness
Walnut leaves	Used in scrofula, herpes and eczema
White wax	White beeswax
Wintergreen	Used as a tea for rheumatism – a similar action to aspirin
Yellow wax	Yellow beeswax
Zinc oleate	Used externally for eczema
Zinc oleostearate	Used externally for eczema and excessive perspiration
Zinc oxide	Used internally for nervous debility, migraine, hysteria. Externally used for skin infections
Zinc phosphide	Nerve stimulant
Zingib.	Zingiber, *see* Ginger

Weights and Measures

Apothecary weights

Apothecary weights were used in Europe for the measurement of pharmaceutical ingredients from as early as 1270. The basis of the apothecary system was the grain. Dispensing and selling were permitted using this system. Weights were as follows.

Apothecary weight				Metric equivalent (g)
gr.	= 1 grain			0.0648
Э	= 1 scruple	= 20 grains		1.2960
ʒ	= 1 drachm	= 60 grains	= 3 scruples	3.8879
℥	= 1 ounce	= 480 grains	= 8 drachms	31.1035
℔	= 1 pound	= 5760 grains	= 12 ounces	393.242

Imperial weights (avoirdupois)

This system, used for the bulk of counter sales, was based on the Imperial pound of 7000 grains, which was subdivided as follows.

Imperial (avoirdupois) weight				Metric equivalent (g)
lb	= 1 pound	= 16 ounces	= 7000 grains	453.5924
oz	= 1 ounce		= 437.5 grains	28.3495

For smaller amounts the ounce was divided into fractions e.g. $^1/_4$ oz, $^1/_2$ oz. Until the end of the 1800s there was also a dram, which was equivalent to one-sixteenth of an ounce or 27.3 grains. The grain weight was the same for both systems.

Imperial measures

Based on the Imperial gallon and subdivided as follows.

Imperial measures			Metric equivalent (ml)
C	= 8 pints		4.54596 litres
O	= 1 pint	= 20 fluid ounces	568.2454
℥	= 1 fluid ounce	= 8 fluid drachms	28.4123
ʒ	= 1 fluid drachm	= 60 minims	3.5515
♏	= 1 minim		0.0592

Metric weights and measures

The metric system of weights is based on the gram (g). A milligram (mg) is one-thousandth of a gram. A kilogram is one thousand grams. Liquid measure is based on the litre (l). A millilitre (ml) is one-thousandth of a litre.

The *British Pharmacopoeia* of 1914 adopted the metric system for all but medicinal doses. Dispensing continued in the apothecary system until 1 January 1971 when metric weights and measures were adopted.

Monetary units

Decimal currency was instigated in the United Kingdom on 15 February 1971. Comparison with the previous monetary system is as follows (equivalents are approximate).

Pre-decimalisation currency		Decimal equivalent (p)
Pound (£)	= 20 shillings	100
Shilling (s)	= 12 pence	5
Penny (d)	= 4 farthings	0.42
Farthing		0.1

The following are examples of written old currency.

£1.10s.6d	One pound, ten shillings and sixpence
1/4d	One shilling and fourpence
£1.1.0	One pound and one shilling (one guinea)
1/1½	One shilling and three halfpence
2/6	Two shillings and sixpence (half a crown)
2/-	Two shillings (a florin)

*I*ndex

Note: Page numbers suffixed with 'f' refer to figures.

H

I

J

K

L

R

rabies (hydrophobia), Dr James on, 90
Radio Luxembourg, Beecham's Pills as sponsor, 25
'Raglan (Field-Marshal Lord)', testimonial to Dalby's Carminative, 65
Raines, Blanshard & Co., Scots Pills and, 14
Raines, Clark & Co. Ltd, Scots Pills and, 14
rectified spirit, 102, 153
red mercuric oxide, 128
Reeves, Elizabeth, testimonial to Zam-Buk, 154, 156-7
Regaine Topical Solution, 10
Reid, George (druggist), 93
resale price maintenance, 7-8
Reynolds (Dr), Dr James's Fever Powder and, 90
Reynolds, Joshua, *The Infant Hercules*, 149
rhubarb, 65, 98, 147
Richards, John Morgan (importer), 44, 139
ringworm, claim for Zam-Buk, 157
Roberts' Alterative Pills, advertisement, 120
Roberts, Giles Lawrence (Dr), inventor of Poor Man's Friend, 117-18
'Robin Hood and Little John' (Devonport, Plymouth), 75
Robinson, Robert E, claim on Dr James's Fever Powder, 90
Roche, Zam-Buk, 159
Rodger, J, Scots Pills and, 14
rooks, Carter's Little Liver Pills, 45
rosin *see* colophony
Royal Holloway College, 80-1
Royal Pharmaceutical Society of Great Britain, 1
    JT Davenport as President, 54
    museum, Scots Pills, 15
    President (1969), on Chlorodyne, 58

S

saffron (crocus), 83, 89
sal volatile, spirit of, 51
sale of PATA-protected goods, 7
sales levels, claimed for Dr James's Fever Powder, 86
salesmen, travelling, Beecham's Pills, 24
salicylate, sodium, 51
Sanitas Company Ltd, Woodward's Gripe Water, 152
saponis *see* soap
sarsaparilla, 52
sassafras oil, 102, 159
Scaffold (singing group), on Pinkham's Vegetable Compound, 109-15
scammony (ipomoea), 33, 35
Schwanberg's powder, 86, 88-9
Science Siftings, on Bile Beans, 31
scientist, fictitious ('Charles Forde'), 28-30
Scots Pills, 13-17, 94
Scott and Bowne, Steedman's Soothing Powders, 132
scrofula
    see also Pilulae Antiscrophulae
Secret Remedies (British Medical Association), 6
    Beecham's Pills, 22, 25-6
    Fennings' Children's Cooling Powders, 69

Singleton's Eye Ointment, 125, 127
Steedman's Soothing Powders, 132
Woodward's Gripe Water, 152
see also More Secret Remedies
Seigel, Edith (inventor of Syrup), 101
Selkirk, G, analysis of Pink Pills for Pale People, 141
semaphore, Beecham's Pills advertisements, 24f
Senate (Canada), GT Fulford on, 139
Senecio aureus (life root), 115
senna, 98, 146, 147
Sentimental and Humorous Essays by G.L. Roberts M.D., 118
Seton Healthcare Group Ltd, 55
Shaker Extract of Roots, 101
Sharp, F (ship's carpenter), testimonial to Beecham's Pills, 24
ships, Browne's inventions, 55
Siam, king Monkut of, Holloway's remedies, 78-9
Singleton, Thomas, Eye Ointment owner, 123-4
Singleton, William (son of Thomas), 124
Singleton's Eye Ointment, 122-8
slogans, Beecham's Pills, 22
Smith Kline & French Co. Inc., Mother Seigel's Syrup, 106
Smith, WF (pharmacist), 131
SmithKline Beecham, 19
soap, 16, 17, 26, 82, 83, 158
    as cholagogue, 33, 35
sodium nuclein, 51
sodium salicylate, 51
sodium tauroglycocholate, 35
soldiers
    Egypt, Singleton's Eye Ointment, 124
    Zam-Buk (claim), 158
    see also army
Somerset House, stamps, Dr James's Fever Powder, 86
song books
    Bile Beans, 31
    published by Thomas Beecham, 22-4
songs
    Beecham's Pills in carol, 27
    Pinkham's Vegetable Compound, 109, 115
Soothing Powders, Steedman's, 129-35
Soothing Syrup, Mrs Winslow's, 143-7
Souter, David (druggist), 93
South, John Arthur, manager of Steedman and Co., 133
spermaceti, 83
spicers, 1
spirit of sal volatile, 51
Squire's Companion, formula for Chlorodyne, 58
St Helens, Thomas Beecham at, 20
St John Ambulance Brigade, 158
St Thomas's Hospital, Holloway's remedies and, 75-6
stamp duty, 5, 9
stamps
    'appropriated', 129
    Dr James's Fever Powder, 86
    proprietary medicines, 5
starch, 44, 133
Stedman's Teething Powders, 133-4
Steedman, John, 129-31
Steedman, Leah (wife of John), 131